THE NEW REIKI MAGIC

The New Reiki Magic

by
Dr. Mohan Makkar
Ph.D. (A.M.)

Winsome Books India

ISBN: 81-88043-10-9

First Edition 2004

© **Dr. Mohan Makkar**
Ph.D. (A.M.)

All rights reserved. No part of this publication may be reproduced or transmitted in any form or by any means, electronic or mechanical, including photocopying, recording, or by any information storage and retrieval system, without permission in writing from the publishers.

Published by
WINSOME BOOKS INDIA
209, F-17, Harsha Complex, Subhash Chowk,
Laxmi Nagar, Delhi-110 092
Email: winsomebooks@rediffmail.com

Printed at : N.H.P. Offset Press, P. Ganj Ind. Area, Delhi-92

Dedicated to:

My Spiritual Guide

**SATCHITANAND SATGURU
SHRI SAINATH MAHARAJ
OF SHIRDI**

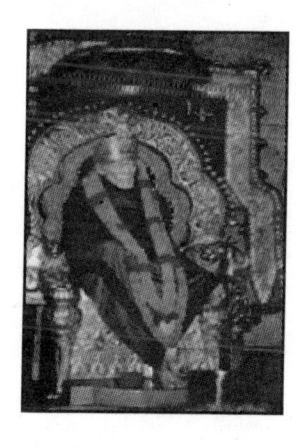

TYPE OF REIKI SYSTEMS PRESENTLY IN USE

The Usui Reiki

Karuna Reiki

Tera Mai Reiki

Brahma Satya Reiki (BSR)

Ryoho (Reiho) Reiki

North of Sixty Reiki

Rainbow Reiki

Hypno Reiki

Sacred Path Reiki

Reiki 4 U

Seichem Reiki

Mystic River Reiki

Omni Reiki

PART I

REIKI 1 - DAY 1

Chapter	Topic discussed	Page No.
1	What is Reiki	1
2	The History of Reiki	4
3	The breathing Technique	10
4	The White Light Meditation	12
5	On Road to Spiritualism	14
6	The 5 Principles of Reiki	15
7	The Reiki Alliance	21
8	On Road to Spiritualism	23
9	Chakras	25
10	The Scanning Technique	34
11	On Road to Spiritualism	35
12	Self-Healing Technique -The hand positions	37
13	Do's & Don'ts about Reiki	43
14	What if you come across cold areas?	44
15	Visual Meditation Exercise - The Glass Technique	45
16	Colours for Health	47
17	The "OM" Meditation	49
18	Summary	50

PART II

REIKI 1 - DAY 2

Chapter	Topic discussed	Page No.
1	Reiki "A" on "B" and "B" on "A"	51
2	Serious Cases - What to do?	62
3	The Reiki Marathon	63
4	Group Healing	65
5	Visual Meditation Exercise - Your Sanctuary	68
6	When not to give REIKI	70
7	Visual Meditation Exercise - Your Counselors	72
8	Visual Meditation Exercise - Your Laboratory	74
9	Meditation	77
10	Reiki - What we have learnt for far	83
11	Questions - Time for Examination	84

PART III

REIKI 2 - DAY 1

Chapter	Topic discussed	Page No.
1	Let's discuss your Self Healing/Reiki Experience	86
2	Why 2nd Degree - a discussion	87
3	On The Roadto Spiritualism	90
4	The Three Reiki Symbols	91
5	What to do with these Symbols?	93
6	Chanting of the Symbols	97
7	Introduction to Mind Control Healing	98
8	The Sound Meditation	104
9	A Medipic Healing Exercise	107
10	Sending Light Healing	108
11	Visual Meditation Exercise - The Universal Bank	109

PART IV

REIKI 2 - DAY 2

Chapter	Topic discussed	Page No.
1	Absentee Healing	111
2	The Short Form of Reiki	113
3	The Reiki Box	115
4	On Road to Spiritualism When Buddhists Meditate	121
5	The Long Form of Reiki	123
6	The Many Faces of Reiki	125
7	Energy Circulation Exercise	127
8	Absentee Healing - Practical Exercise	128
9	Visual Meditation Exercise - Let's Travel	129
10	Activating your Ethereal Body	132
11	The Yin & The Yang Pain Killers	134
12	The Yin & The Yang - Method of Healing	138
13	Summary	140

PART V

REIKI 3A - THE MASTER'S DEGREE

Chapter	Topic discussed	Page No.
1	A discussion	142
2	What is Reiki 3A	144
3	The Master Symbol	145
4	Do you need Regression?	147
5	Do you live by the Attitude of Gratitude way of life?	149
6	Questions & Answers	152

PART VI

REIKI 3B - THE MASTER/TEACHER

Chapter	Topic discussed	Page No.
1	Preparing for an attunement	154
2	The Technique - Attunement Reiki	155
3	Meditation 20 minutes	164
4	What we have learnt so far	166
5	Problems & Problems	167
6	What to do and what not to do	170
7	Visual Mediation Exercise - The Balloon & The Stones	171
8	Meditation 20 minutes	172
9	What if no results follow?	173
10	The Positive & the Negative Mind	175
11	Why is a Certificate Necessary?	177
12	Let's Sum Up	178
13	The Presentation of the Certificates	179
14	How to Close each day	180
15	Questions	181
16	Just to Say Good-Bye	184
17	The Human Anatomy	185
18	Diseases & Hand Positions for Treatments	186

ACKNOWLEDGEMENTS

First and foremost to Mother Mahashakti resident in my Crown Chakra, The Archangels, The Seven Princes, My Higher Self, My Spiritual Guide, The Reiki Spirit which is always present during the teaching & healing practices and through which miraculously serious cases have been healed. Not to forget the Reiki Light.

My Gurus Dr. Pradeep Diwan, Dr. Geeta for the love and light. The light in me would have been sucked away long ago, had it not been for their power to let me remain in this world to serve.

Thanks to all my students for giving me their time and love and accepting me as their Guru/Master. Thanks to all my patients who have given me a chance to treat and heal them, and, be one with them for a few stations in the journey of life.

Thanks to the media Gulf News & ARY.

Thanks to all of you who have come and gone silently as the breath does not knowing it is giving life every precious moment.

With love and light

Dr. Mohan Makkar Ph.D. (A.M.)

SPECIAL THANKS TO:

- ✝ Tejal for "Self Healing" Photographs.
- ✝ Tejal & Harsh for the Reiki 'A' on 'B' photographs.

- ✝ Bharat & Monica - my Master Level Students who have explained the Attunement Technique of Usui Shiki Ryoho.

REIKI 1

DAY 1

INTRODUCTION

Welcome to Reiki Class 1. Let me introduce myself. I am your Reiki Teacher. My name is Dr. Mohan Makkar, I have completed my Ph.D. from the Alternative Medicines College in Calcutta which is affiliated with Russia and USA. Before we proceed further I would like to tell you how I was introduced to **REIKI "THE UNIVERSAL HEALING ENERGY"**

For the past few years I have been treating people by 'absentee healing' method, an art that is hereditary and partially acquired through my father.

The main problem I faced while healing people was, unconsciously, I took the disease of the sick people on myself. The results were always positive, people were healed, but I remained sick most of the time. So much so, that my wife and children got fed up of my sickness.

Pressure started building up. Finally, the lid blew up and I got a notice from my wife "I have had enough, either you choose treating the sick people or you choose me, I will not let you have both!" I was in a dilemma. I strongly believe that nature takes it's own course, and, in my case it did.

I met a girl named Manjusha. She contacted me for her mother who had 'frozen shoulders'. I treated her mother and Manjusha thanked me personally. At this time she declared that she was a Reiki Master herself. What is REIKI? I asked her. She explained to me.

I poured out my grievances to her. She suggested that I should go for a Reiki Course. I did attend the Reiki Course. Rciki 1 was through a teacher - who got me, really fooled. I believe she is just a Reiki Master not a Reiki Master/Teacher. Attunements were given by the Reiki Master and I believed that I had the power to heal without taking the illnesses on myself, till the time I came across another Reiki Master/Teacher.

I went for a refresher course with the new Reiki Master/Teacher and while doing the advance Reiki course (Reiki 2), he told me that my palms were not becoming warm, as they should. This is the time when he asked me how the attunements were given. I explained to him, and, he laughed. I knew that sarcastic laugh and understood that somewhere I had been cheated.

I paid the course fee of Reiki 1 and Reiki 2 to this Reiki Master/Teacher and started practicing the new healing technique on my patients, physically and in absentia. At this juncture let me point out, that I mixed my own techniques with the Reiki Method and the results were superb.

I have treated cases like Asthma, paralysis, Arthritis, Cough and Colds, tooth aches, Conjunctivitis, Diabetes, Rheumatism, Spondilitis, Migraine, Memory lapses, Brain Tumor, lung Collapse, Comatic cases, with astounding success. Presently, I am treating cases of, Blood Plasma, Diabetes, Asthma, Severed Cornea, migraine, Vertigo, Lumbago, etc.

I have stopped remaining sick. The sicknesses of other people do not harm my health any more. I teach during the weekends and have witnessed the transformation of my students. I do not claim every student of mine has had a transformation. Actually, the results they get depend on the efforts they put in

The more you practice, the more you gain. Nobody sees you, but remember you are your own judge and you will witness your own failings and your own success. Be true and honest to yourself and you shall succeed. That is my promise.

During the complete course of Reiki - taking you gradually through to Reiki Master/Teacher's degree, we shall do some Visual Meditation Exercises and learn the art of Meditation also. We shall also touch on the topics of other healing techniques and discuss some of them.

For the visual meditation exercises, a technique of breathing will be taught to you, which you have to constantly practice & master.

Also, the secret symbols will be given to you and the art of attuning with easy to follow illustrations will be taught to you step by step.

A question may arise in your mind, that there are dozens of books written on Reiki, so why another? Why this book? Without egoism I state that the idea of writing a UNIQUE BOOK on REIKI was given to me and I thought of writing it in a classroom format. How far I have succeeded in this effort it is for you to decide.

This introduction can go on endlessly, but I will end here with a brief thought:

It is wisely said:

***YOU DON'T HAVE TO GO TO THE SEA AND WAIT,
TO CATCH THE FISH, AT LEAST, YOU HAVE TO PUT IN THE
BAIT.***

Like a well, the more Reiki energy you use, the more you will get, HAVE HAPPY REIKI-ING hours and wishing you A PERFECT HEALTH.

DR. MOHAN MAKKAR PH.D. (A.M.)

REIKI 1

DAY 1
CHAPTER 1

WHAT IS REIKI?

Have you read any book on Reiki?

There are many books available on this subject. The descriptions, the history, the principles are always the same. The story of Dr. Usui Mikao cannot be changed; neither can the characters of Dr. Hayashi or Mrs. Takata.

Do you know that Reiki is made up of two syllables "REI" & "KI".

"REI" stands for "UNIVERSAL" and
"KI" stands for "ENERGY"

This explanation is best given in the book "Reiki" written by Bodo & Shalila, which is as follows:

This Universal Energy has existed amidst us from the beginning of the Universe. Thousands of years ago the Tibetans already possessed a deep understanding of the nature of spirit, energy and matter. They used this knowledge to heal their bodies, harmonize their souls and lead their spirits to an experience of unity.

This knowledge was guarded and preserved by the mystery schools and was available to a very few people, usually priests or spiritual leaders who in turn passed this technique to their disciples by word of mouth.

The knowledge of Reiki would have remained lost forever had not Dr. Mikao Usui rediscovered the key, which led to the recovery of a thousand-year old tradition of healing in 2500-year-old Sanskrit sutras at the end of the 19th century.

Reiki - the Universal Energy is defined as being that power which acts and lives in all created matter.

The Usui system of Reiki is not only the most simple and natural healing method we know of, but it is also the most effective way of transferring this universal life energy. Once the attunements are given to a person he becomes a Reiki Channel and will remain so for the rest of his life.

We will mostly be talking about this Universal Life Energy, which is the base of our classes = REIKI.

The human body consists of about 100 billion (100,000,000,000,000) cells. These cells in turn possess about 100,000 differing genes, consisting of long, spiral-formed DNA chains. Every single one of these microscopically small cells contains within itself no less than the total genetic construction plans for our bodies.

If we were to roll out all these spiraled chains and join them up, their length would amount to more than 120 billion kilometers, about 800 times the distance between the earth and the sun. And yet all these chains of DNA molecules would fit into the size of a walnut.

Just think the greatness of the energy that all these forms of life manifest. How great must be the intelligence which gives these forms of life shape and structure. The question that rises in our midst is that: did our universe and our lives arise out of a chain of coincidences, as a materialistic view of things would have us believe? Can unconscious matter bring forth consciousness? Can it bring forth the spirit? The Soul? Even scientists are baffled by these queries. The result is same-That a superior intelligent force DOES EXIST. A Universal Spirit, which is continually creating the universe out of itself.

Super gravitation theory describes the existence of a standardized, perfectly balanced field standing in relationship to only itself, a field of pure intelligence, which brings forth all matter to form the basis of all creation. Wise man often tell the stories that in a state of being contains all creation and out of which all life arose. The energy of this state of being lives in all things, and it is this universal energy, which flows through our hands in concentrated form when we treat someone with Reiki.

In short it means - Reiki has a holistic effect. It reaches all levels of existence and strives to bring these differing levels into a state of balance. The therapist is only a channel of energy, because it is not his own energy, which passes through his hands, but it is a Universal Energy, which leaves the Reiki Channel strengthened and harmonized. This universal energy seems to have a mind of it's own, for it knows how much and where the person needs the energy. It is not for us do decide or in our control to add or subtract this energy.

Reiki is experienced as love. This love is a power, which unites us to a state of oneness with the whole of creation. Love is the original home of the soul.

Reiki is the healing method in the broadest sense of the word. For it not only heals the body, but the spiritual self also. Reiki has nothing to do with religion, spiritualism, occult in any shape or form. Neither it is hypnotic or any other psychological technique.

An atheist can practice Reiki too, by the positive thinking people and the negative thinking people.

Today the rediscovery of Reiki has set forth a trend of healing technique where no medicines are instilled in the body of the patient, no prayers are mumbled, yet the results are achieved.

Reiki attunements bring forth the developments in you, which have been dormant, and you become a better person.

REIKI 1

DAY 1
CHAPTER 2

THE HISTORY OF REIKI

The ancient healing method of Reiki was re-discovered in the middle of the nineteenth century by Dr. Mikao Usui, who was also responsible for its revival.

Dr. Mikao Usui - August 15, 1865 - March 9, 1926

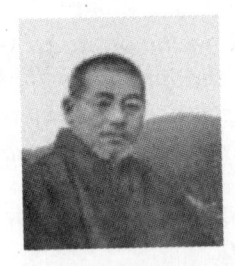

The story of Dr. Usui's search for this secret knowledge has been told by Grand Master Hawayo Takata (1900-1980) along the following lines:

Mikao Usui was the Dean of a Christian College in Kyoto, Japan. One day, some of his pupils asked him why they had nothing of the healing methods used by Jesus Christ and whether Dr. Usui would be able to carry out such a healing for them. Since he was unable to answer these questions, Dr. Usui decided to resign from his position as per the Japanese customs.

He decided to study Christianity in a Christian country until he found the answers to the questions posed to him by his students.

His journey led him to America, where he attended the University of Chicago and became a Doctor of Theology. However, he could not find a satisfactory answer in Christian writings and, not having found one in Chinese scriptures either, he traveled to North India, where he was able to study the Holy Writings. Dr. Usui had not only the knowledge of Japanese, Chinese and English languages, but he also became a master of Sanskrit language.

He later returned to Japan, where he discovered some Sanskrit formulas and symbols in old Buddhist sutras, which seemed to hold the answers to his questions. At the time, he was living a monastery in Kyoto, and, after he had spoken to the Head, he set off to the Holy Mountain of Kuriyama, which lay 16 miles away. Here he intended to fast and meditate in solitude for 21 days in the hope of gaining contact with the level of consciousness the Sanskrit symbols had been written on in order to determine the truth of their contents.

Once he reached at the top of the mountain, he laid 21 pebbles in front of him and removed one at the passing of each day as a kind of calendar. During this time, he read the Sutras, sang and meditated. Nothing unusual happened until the last day dawned. It was still quite dark when he saw a small shining light moving towards him with great speed. He tried to get up and run, but as an after thought he stayed put. The light became bigger and bigger and finally hit him in the middle of his forehead - the 3rd eye Chakra. Dr. Usui's thoughts were that he was going to die when he suddenly saw millions of little bubbles in blue, lilac, pink and all the colours of the rainbow. Then he saw a great white light, and the well-known Sanskrit symbols in front of him glowing in shining gold and he muttered "Yes, I remember" before he fell unconscious.

This was the birth of Reiki.

When Dr. Usui Mikao returned to the normal state of consciousness, the sun had already arisen. Though he had had a complete fast for 21 days, he was surprised to find that he felt full of strength and energy. He began to descend the mountain. In his rush, he stubbed his toe. Blood started flowing from the toe. Reflexively he covered the toe with the palm of his hand and much to his surprise the bleeding stop and after a few moments the pain vanished. This was the first miracle.

Since he was hungry, he stopped at an inn and ordered a large Japanese breakfast. For those who do not know about Japanese breakfast, it can be stated that a single large Japanese breakfast can be easily shared with a friend or two who have good appetites. The *innkeeper saw Dr. Usui's clothes and his beard, and, knew he had been fasting. He requested Dr. Usui to have a soup and something light. But, Dr. Usui refused. He did intake the complete Japanese breakfast without any side effects. This was the second miracle.*

The innkeeper's granddaughter who served the food to him was suffering for a bad toothache. Her mouth was swollen. Dr. Usui asked the innkeeper if he could treat the child. The innkeeper somehow knew that his guest was no ordinary person. He gave Dr. Usui the permission. As soon as Dr. Usui laid his hands on the girl's cheeks, the pain vanished and after a few minutes the swelling also subsided. This was the third miracle.

Dr. Usui returned to the monastery, where his friend the abbot was lying in bed, suffering from arthritis. Dr. Usui sat besides him and placed his hands on the abbot. The abbot started feeling better and was mobile after a short period.

Dr. Usui decided to go to the Beggars City in the slums of Kyoto, treat the beggars and help them lead a better life. He spent seven years in the asylum, treating many diseases. One day, however, he saw the same faces. On querying why they kept coming back, he got the answer that begging was a better way of life than taking the burden of getting married and raising children and having a routine job.

Dr. Usui was deeply shaken and wept. He knew that he had greatly forgotte something important - namely : to teach the beggars gratitude. In the following days he thought out some Reiki maxims – <u>The 5 principles of Reiki</u>

Soon afterwards Dr. Usui left the asylum and returned to Kyoto, where he kindled a large torch and stood in the streets. Asked for the reason by the passers-by, Dr. Usui told them he was looking for people in search of the true Light, people who were ill oppressed and who were longing to be healed. This was the beginning of his new gift, which he spent traveling around and teaching Reiki.

Dr. Usui gave up his body. Dr. Usui is now buried in a Kyoto temple, with the story of his life written on his gravestone. It is said that the Emperor of Japan honored his grave.

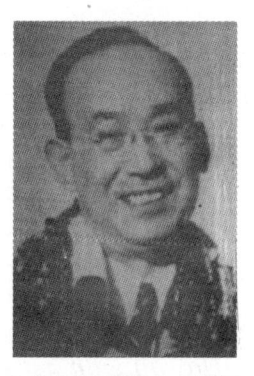

DR. CHUJIRO HAYASHI - c.1878 - May 9, 1940

One of Dr. Usui's closest collaborators, Dr. Chijiro Hayashi, took his place, becoming the second Reiki Grand Master in the line of tradition. He ran a private Reiki Clinic in Tokyo until 1940, where unusually severe cases could be treated, with Reiki being applied "round the clock" in the event of especially serious illnesses. Frequently a patient would also receive Reiki from several practitioners at once. The effects of the Second World War and the death of Dr. Hayashi on 10th May 1941 put an end to his work.

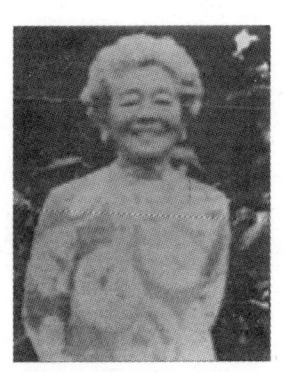

Mrs. Hawayo Takata
December 24, 1900 - December 11, 1980

Mrs. Hawayo Takata became Dr. Huyashi's successor. She was born in 1900 on the island of Hawaii as the child of Japanese parents but was a citizen of the United States. She was a widow with two small children, She was suffering from a number of severe illnesses at the time when an inner voice told her to go to Japan and seek healing there.

Having arrived in Japan, she was lying on the operating table, about to undergo an operation, when the voice spoke to her again, telling her that the operation was unnecessary. She asked her doctor about other methods of treatment and he advised her to go to Dr. Hayashi's Reiki clinic. Once there, she was applied Reiki daily by two practitioners and, after a few months, she had won back her health completely.

Hawayo Takata became a pupil of Dr. Hayashi for a period of one year and then returned to Hawaii with her daughters. Dr. Hayashi made her a Reiki Master when he visited Hawaii in 1938. On his death in 1941, she succeeded him as the Grand Master. She lived and healed in Hawaii for many years, but she first began to train Reiki Masters herself when she was in her seventies. On 11, December 1980, Hawayo Takata passed away, leaving 22 Reiki Grand Masters in the USA and Canada.

Today there are hundreds of thousands Reiki Master/Teachers in the world. References of teachers in countries/cities is easily available on the website.

Mrs. Takata's 22 Grand Masters.

George Araki

Dorothy Baba

Ursula Baylow

Rick Bockner

Patricia Bowling

Barbara Brown

Fran Brown

Phyllis Furumoto

Beth Gray

John Gray

Iris Ishikuro

Harry Kuboi

Ethel Lombardi

Barbara McCullough

Mary McFadyen

Paul Mitchell

Bethel Phaigh

Shinobu Saito

Virginia Samdahl

Wanja Twan

Barbara Weber Ray

Kay Yamashita

REIKI 1

DAY 1
CHAPTER 3

THE BREATHING TECHINIC

Importance Of Breathing
There are two reasons why breathing is important. (1) To supply our bodies and its various organs with oxygen which is important for our survival and (2) to get rid of waste products and toxins from the body.

Importance of Healthy Breathing
Breathing comes to us automatically, unconsciously and naturally. Breathing occurs all the time, though we are unaware of it. As no one teaches us to breathe, we begin to breathe sluggishly, assume slouched positions which diminish lung capacities and short breaths. Moreover, the rising pollution level globally does not help our respiratory system. Yes, one more thing, Mental tensions, stress, anger, deep thoughts can produce restricted breathing.

What's Wrong With The Way We Breathe?
Our breath is too shallow and quick. We do not take enough oxygen and thus eliminate CO_2, resulting in starvation of O_2 in our bodies. Remember, every cell in the body needs O_2 and our level of energy and rejuvenation is just a product of the health of all the cells.

Healthy lungs require deep breathing, so they can function 100% and our vitality too is 100%.

THE TECHNIQUE

Let's learn the breathing technique. This breathing exercise will help you to centralize your thoughts and keep your mind from wandering, whilst curing innumerable diseases like Allergies, Asthma, Migraines, heart, lungs, stomach, liver problems etc.

Step 1 - Take a deep breath in from your nose to your navel chord (belly button) to the count of 4. Inflate your stomach as much as possible while breathing in. Breathe in with me 1...2...3...4 - STOP.

Step 2 - Hold your breath to the count of 4: 1.... 2.... 3.... 4
Step 3 - Now breathe out slowly through your mouth, 1.... 2.... 3...4 deflate your stomach as you breathe out.
Step 4 - Hold your breath to the count of 4.

Continue the same till you feel completely relaxed or slightly dizzy.

What happens is this:

From the time we are born to the time we depart this world we breathe. But, nobody teaches us how to breathe. What we do is we swim in the swallow waters; we never go into the deep. In between the thorax and trunk there are no bones. There are only floating ribs. These ribs survive on air. If we do not breathe in properly, we start to curl up. You may have seen cases of elderly people who curl up as the age increases.

What we have to do is, breathe in deeply through the nose, until feel the air go to the navel. Hold the breathe in there to the count of 4, and then release the breath through the mouth.

12 sets in the morning, 12 sets in the afternoon and 12 sets late evening, will work wonders. For instance, those small ailments, like Sinus, Coughs & Cold, Memory Lapses, Headaches, Migraines, Body aches, Allergies, Asthmatic attacks, will be cured. You will feel the difference yourself. So, why not start now?

(Care has to be taken not to overdo any of the exercises that are being taught to you. A correct dose of anything will help you maintain your health, but an over dose of anything can ruin your health. So, please take care to do and follow what is being specified.)

Note: Not recommended for patients with Heart Problems

REIKI 1

DAY 1
CHAPTER 4

THE WHITE LIGHT MEDITATION

A VISUAL MEDITATIONAL EXERCISE

In every Reiki Class, we do a Meditation known as the "White Light Meditation". During this Meditation, we heal the world by sending a flow of positive energy to make our world a better place to live in.

- Do your breathing exercise as taught to you. (4 breaths in, 4 hold, 4 out & 4 hold - repeat) - only 3 or maximum 4 sets. We will call this CENTRALISING for future records.

- Now, on an out breath, with your mental power create a white ball, the size of a tennis ball. Make this ball spin clockwise with your mental power of visualisation. Visualize it; see it with your mental eyes in front of your third eye Chakra, the center of your eyebrows. See it spin, slow….slow….slow, now it is picking up speed fast…fast….faster…faster.

- As the speed is increasing, visualize a white light emitting from the ball, this white light is like a mist, a fog. See the white light cover the ball. The amazing thing you notice is that this white light is floating and covering you and the furniture in the room. Repeat see it like a haze, a mist. See it cover the room.

- Let this light float into the other rooms, the kitchen, the bathroom, the storeroom, the bedroom and all the other rooms in your apartment. Now, extend your vision, see it seep out of the balcony doors, the windows, and the main door and visualize it going out into the street. Visualize the white light covering your building.

- The speed of the white light is increasing. The white light is now covering the area in which you live. See the white light cover the town, the city you live in.

- See the white light cover the other surrounding cities.

- See the white light cover the entire nation. The white light is now covering surrounding nations and the full world.

- Visualize the white light cover all the mentally handicapped children. See the children improving under the influence of this WHITE LIGHT. See them becoming better and better and better. See the white light cover all the pregnant women. Visualize the pregnant women delivering healthy children normally. Visualize the white light cover the people with terminal diseases like Cancer and Aids. See these people recovering. Visualize the white light cover all the undernourished children on this planet. Visualize these children eating lavishly. See the recovering gradually and learning to smile. Visualize the while light covers all the prisons in this world Visualize the prisoner's turn into better humans.

- Visualize the world leaders signing a peace treaty under the white light.

- Visualize the terrorist's throw up their arms and surrender them.

- Visualize brotherhood and love floating in every heart in every being. Visualize all politicians turning to new leaves and working for the benefit of mankind. Keep this visualisation in the level of your 3rd eye chakra.

Slowly come back to the room and open your eyes whenever you feel like it.

At this time I will take a short break.

Why don't you also relax for 5 minutes? Have a nice cup of hot tea/coffee or sip a cold juice, before we go into our main subject - REIKI.

REIKI 1

DAY 1
CHAPTER 5

ON THE ROAD TO SPIRITUALISM

- *"Water in lakes, pits, wells and rivers is rain water, though the taste, color, name and form are different, based on where the rain has fallen and how pure the container is. Divine grace is like rain, pure, pellucid, falling on all. How it is received and used depends on the individual"*

- *"When you have done your best and that is found not enough, then call on me. I am ever ready to reinforce your exertions with my grace"*

- *"Generally, the avatar (the coming) is described as a 'coming down' from a higher status to a lower one. But no! When the baby in the cradle weeps, wails and clamors for help, the mother stoops and takes it in her arms. Her stoop is not to be described as a 'coming down.'"*

REIKI 1

DAY 1
CHAPTER 6

THE 5 PRINCIPALS OF REIKI

When. Dr. Usui was deeply shaken on finding out the beggars was returning to the beggar City; he knew that he had forgotten to teach them gratitude. In his solace, he thought of the following maxims, which are today known as "THE 5 PRINCIPLES OF REIKI"

1. *JUST FOR TODAY, I WILL LIVE THE ATTITIDE OF GRATITUDE.*
2. *JUST FOR TODAY, I WILL NOT WORRY*
3. *JUST FOR TODAY, I WILL NOT ANGER*
4. *JUST FOR TODAY, I WILL EARN MY LIVING HONESTLY*
5. *JUST FOR TODAY, I WILL HONOUR MY PARENTS, TEACHERS & ELDERS.*

1. <u>JUST FOR TODAY, I WILL LIVE THAT ATTITUDE OF GRATITUDE..</u>

To live in gratitude is to live in abundance. When we are constantly in the attitude of gratitude state, feeling thankful not only for what we have received but for what we know and trust will constantly be provided, we being to magnetically attract abundance. Our normal state is that of abundance. It is only our connection with the race mind consciousness (or collective unconscious) of lack, and our own conditioning, which keeps us from accepting that which is truly ours.

One of the fundamental concepts at the root of the major philosophical and religious systems in ancient times was that of all sufficiency. It was taught that to understand one's self was to understand God that by going deep within, one could transmute fear into love, ignorance into wisdom, and lack into abundance.

Jesus said, "…what you see you shall be" In other words, if you focus on what you do not have, you will continue to be in lack. On the other hand, if you continue to be aware of the unlimited abundance all around you, and constantly feel the resulting gratitude, abundance will continue to be your state of affairs, and even increase. There is nothing lacking on this planet, it is the distribution system that has gone haywire due to our illusions about lack, not to mention man's greed, due again, to fear of lack, that has indeed kept us in lack.

To be in gratitude is to know at the core of your being that all is one, that separation is an illusion. Another important factor is to be able to accept the abundance that is rightfully ours. If we feel subconsciously "unworthy" of the riches and wealth of the Universe, we will block the flow of abundance to us. Many people now suffer from this consciousness of separation from the Absolute - that which embodies all that is. The long history of guilt of separation from the Absolute, keep even those people who seem to follow and live in accord with the laws of Universal harmony, away from the true success and prosperity which is rightfully theirs. The casual factor must be sought in each individual.

In most cases, the channels through which affluence and harmony normally flow are either developed or paralyzed. Universal Life Energy must then be used in order to give to those channels their natural functions. Once this connection is made, success and prosperity will be obtained. In the realm of the Absolute, every action, every cause, results in a perfect effect, which is complete success. The only reason that most people do not achieve it is because they are not aligned with it, or are closed to it.

2. *JUST FOR TODAY, I WILL NOT WORRY:*

To worry is to forget that there is a divine or universal purpose to everything. It we are truly in tune with the guidance of our higher-selves, and live each day to the best of our ability, we are then aware that we have done everything in our power that we possible can, and the rest is up to the Universal Life Force. Worry is a thought pattern, which results from a feeling of separateness from the "I AM" consciousness. To worry about the past is futile - we must remember that each person, including ourselves, does the best that he can in each of life's situations, in accordance with the knowledge or wish he has at any given moment. We are all products of our conditioning and tend to reach accordingly. If we regret a past action of ours; realise that we reacted according to our resources; then we should be thankful for the lesson and move on. At the same time, realise that others did all injustices done to us in the past as a result of their conditioning. We can only wish them well and hope that they too have learned from their actions.

To worry after the future is also futile. It is said "Expect the best in life, and, when you receive something that you didn't expect, acknowledge that it is the best for you in your present situation" Even if what occurs seems very negative at the time, it is only a lesson. Somehow, we helped create that situation, even if on a subconscious level, to learn. So feel gratitude that it has come to pass, and that we are free; then move on. Surrender, to the Higher Self, and try not to interfere with the Universal timing in life. Know that in our perfect flow there is a synchronicity of events, as long as we have completed our part in the scheme of things, all else will be taken care of. Worrying results from illogical and irrational patterns of thought, creating in turn more limitations and a further separation in consciousness. We should surrender today to our Higher-Self's plan and release ourselves from worry.

3. *JUST FOR TODAY, I WILL NOT ANGER:*

Anger, in reality, is a totally unnecessary emotion. Like most inappropriate reactive emotions, it has its roots in the feeling of guilt from having separated ourselves from the Universal Consciousness. To anger is to desire no control, which results from feeling out of control, indeed out of synchronization with our divine or universal life purpose. Many people allowed their ego to direct their life course, at the same time ignoring the inner guidance, which would otherwise lead them to a natural and harmonious flow. By allowing the ego to be effected by inappropriate desires and expectations, we suffer untold grief.

When our expectations get the best of us, and we become angry, because someone didn't live up to our needs and desires, we tend to forget that those we have drawn into our environment are only our mirrors. Every thought that we think sets up a cause, and the effect may come back when we least expect it. Truly, every situation is a mirror, a direct reflection of cause and effect, created by us. Those who happen to "press our buttons" or stimulate our weak points, are not really the cause of our anger. They are there to learn as well. We drew each other in a mutual need to complete certain lessons. When someone spurs us on to anger, we should try to stop the emotion, (refer the art of living) by observing our reactions to others and ourselves and become more consciously aware of our reactions, and, in time, master our emotions. We should also feel gratitude for having been given the opportunity to witness our weak points, as only growth can result.

Ultimately, if we do get angry, we should not feel guilty for experiencing that anger. It has been programmed into us for so many generations, that it is difficult at first not to be triggered when we are "attacked" by the anger of others. In addition, we have long allowed our expectations to get the best of us, and tend to take things personally when things don't go our way.

The hurt feelings, which result, cause us to blast out in anger. While attempting to "reprogram our old anger tapes", we must allow ourselves to release our emotions, and not hold anger in. What we can do is tone down our reactions by expressing, in a calm way, how someone's negative statement makes us feel. If the other person persists in a loud way, it is wise to leave their vicinity and regain our power by not reacting. The best action to take, in the beginning of any episode, is not to react, but to emanate love. It is difficult to feel anger while we are smiling. Our smile may even trigger a "mirror effect" in the other person.

Finally, anger is a very disharmonious energy, which creates disease in the body. It would be of great benefit to learn to transform this energy by dealing with it constructively. Just for today do not anger - be in attitude of gratitude.

4. *JUST FOR TODAY I WILL EARN MY LIVING HONESTLY:*

Of great importance to a harmonious life flow is honesty in dealing with oneself. To be honest with oneself is to face the truth in all things. Many of us live in a fantasy world when it comes to perceiving reality. When we deny the truth about reality and are ultimately faced with truth, we may become severely disjointed. Sometimes the truth seems hard to deal with in our world, but if we look deeply, examine our own behavior, and discover the purposes that various people and situations have in our lives, we will develop compassion for all.

To live in trust is to be aligned with our Higher Self's purpose. Living in truth is also the simplest, least complex way to live. Truth brings clarity. When we face life honestly, we can see more clearly the lessons we are here to learn, and complete them with much less effort. Living a life of illusion is much more complex. Denial then takes a center focus, and soon a web of falsehood may so thoroughly bind us, to "protect" us from the truth, that we may have difficulty finding our way out of the maze.

If we are honest with ourselves, we will tend to project honesty onto others. It then becomes easy to "do unto others as you would have others do unto you". When we do our work honestly, we are being truthful to our Higher Self. This truth is reinforced by love for others, and ourselves, which helps to create harmony in our life. So, let's live in truth vitalized by love, and just for today do our work honestly.

5. *JUST FOR TODAY, I WILL HONOUR MY PARENTS, TEACHERS & ELDERS*

Truly, we are all of one source. It is also clear that all forms of life are interdependent. The destructive changes that have occurred in recent times on the planet, (which have happened as a result of Man's insensitivity to the delicate ecological balance); have opened us up to this fact. In order to survive, we are discovering that we will have to drop our self-centred tendency to want to control nature, and learn to show love and respect for all life forms.

Through the study of physics, we now know that we are all a collective energy from the same source. There is truly no solid matter, only different levels of vibrations. All forms of matter vibrate at different energy levels, yet they are all interconnected, because there are not solid barriers between them. Thus when we accept all of the various aspects of ourselves, it affects all others. Likewise, when we accept others, we too feel the reflection in ourselves. As a result, any positive energy, whether directed at others, or ourselves helps to heal the whole planet. Each person, animal, plant and mineral is included in the whole. To show love and respect to all others is to love and respect ourselves and our mother earth, so, just for today, show love and respect for every living being.

REIKI 1

DAY 1
CHAPTER 7

THE REIKI ALLIANCE

Just before the demise of Grand Master Mrs. Hawayo Takata on 11th December, 1980, Mrs. Takata and some of the Reiki Masters grounded in August, 1980 the American Reiki Association which was to organise and co-ordinate the passing on of the knowledge of Reiki.

Today, Reiki s represented by two Organizations which have succeeded the first and which are both based in the USA, One has been The American International Reiki Association Inc., ·(The A.I.R.A. now called the T.R.T.A.I.) and the other is THE REIKI ALLIANCE.

The Reiki Alliance was founded in 1981 by Phyllis Lee Furumoto, the grand daughter of Mrs. Hawayo Takata, and a ground of 21 Reiki Masters, in the form of an open association. The "Reiki Alliance" was registered in the USA as a non-profit organization in 1981, with Phyllis Lee Furumoto holding the position of the Grand Master. At the beginning of 1987, about 100 Reiki Masters, some of them living in Europe, were members of the Alliance. Most of the Masters trained by Hawayo Takata belong to this organization. The Reiki Alliance takes a spiritual approach to the spreading of Reiki and keeps to the traditional teachings. The Alliance is of the opinion that the Truth finds its way to the hearts of those open and prepared for it and, therefore, they rarely advertise.

The AMERICAN INTERNATIONAL REIKIA ASSOCIATION Inc. (A.I.R.A.) was found in 1982, by Dr. Barbara Weber Ray, Dr. Ray had also been trained by Hawayo Takata to convey the knowledge involved in the attainment of the Master grade to others and became the President of this group. The A.I.R.A. has been concerned with research into scientific aspects of Reiki to a large extent and is known for its well-organized publicity efforts. It has founded a Reiki documentation center and carries out symposiums, conferences and exhibitions and is active in public events. The Association also trains teachers of Reiki.

We are of the opinion that both complement each other in their efforts to teach and spread the idea of Reiki. If a feeling arises that you should join one of them, search your heart, rely on your intuition and join the organization that best answers your needs.

REIKI 1

DAY 1
CHAPTER 8

ON THE ROAD TO SPIRITUALISM

A Lecture: (An Elementary observation/exercise)

"Just have one awareness when you cross the road. Develop the awareness that you are crossing the road. When you are walking, you will not be noting lifting, forward and placing in the middle of the road. Before you go into the kitchen, you bring one awareness to your mind 'going into the kitchen.' You do not need to do the naming exercise.

"However, try to produce direct awareness of what you are doing without saying anything mentally. We do naming in intensive practice only. Naming will come to an end at a certain level even in intensive practice. It is just like using a raft to cross a river. Once you are on the other side, you do not need the raft or boat or anymore. Naming is just a raft. The technique is just a raft used to cross to the other side.

"When you are going to work, bring about one awareness in the mind 'going to work.' When you are going to drive 'going to drive.' In case you have to drive continuously for a few hours, often bring in an awareness that you are behind the wheel. You come to a traffic jam, there should be one awareness 'traffic jam.' Make yourself aware of it as soon as possible. Make yourself aware of it as soon as possible. If you do not have that awareness, you may forget that you are sharing the road with other people. If you want to go quickly, you may want other vehicles out of your way so unreasonably that you create agitation in yourself. So when you are behind the wheel, have just one awareness, 'you are behind the wheel'

"You go to the supermarket and have picked up many things. In front of ;you is a long queue. Retain the awareness 'a long queue'. This will sustain your ability to be patient. Otherwise, you will be standing in the queue feeling miserable. We spend many years of our lives in anxiety, worry, frustration and fear. How nice it would be if we could reduce these negative emotions that take away our ability to enjoy life. We will then have more good times.

"You go to work as a doctor and see so many patients in the surgery. You allow yourself to make a conscious awareness by observing 'many patients.' Otherwise, you will come under pressure unconsciously. This will cause you work-stress. You have to finish your work by lunchtime but more patients keep coming. The pressure keeps building up.

"Suppose, you go into your office. Someone comes to work with a disturbed mind maybe having had some problems at home. You are not sure what he has been through for the last few hours. What you should is to be aware of the fact that you are in the office with others, and, you are not at home, where things are at your disposal. It is a different environment. This prepares you to face something uncertain. You would not take things for granted as you do at home. If you see someone speaking very impolitely or in a stressful manner, you have to observe him as 'being stressful."

PART 1

DAY 1
CHAPTER 9

CHAKRAS

AFTER BREAKFAST:

All were seated.

"In approximately 2,465 techniques in Alternative Medicine world some words keep on re-occurring, viz. Auras, Chakras, the 7 bodies etc. Let's begin with the Chakras."

"Chakras & Auras"

"Chakras are the psychic centres in the body that are active at all times, whether we are conscious of them or not. Energy moves through the chakras to produce difference psychic states. Modern biological science explains this as the chemical changes produced by the endocrine glands, ductless glands whose secretions mix into the body's bloodstream directly and instantaneously.

"Ancient philosophers of the East related those changes with the five basic elements viz. Earth, Water, Fire, Air and Ether.

"Knowledge about the Chakras can be a valuable key to introspection. It is possible to observe oneself and see energy moving through the various psychic centres. Religious practices such as fasting, charity and selfless service cause the energy to flow into the higher centres;

The dormant energy coiled in the "root chakra" becomes active and begins its ascent. After the flow has reached the higher centres, the total attitude of the practitioner changes; this feeling is referred to repeatedly as a new birth.

Maintaining the upward flow of energy then becomes the primary concern of such a person. The constant, simultaneous practice of visualization and recitation of mantras help the aspirant to maintain the flow of energy in higher centres and thus gets beyond the elements.

"Chakras are basics to the awakening of the Kundalini. But, in Reiki, the sole purpose of studying the chakras is to give more energy to these chakras to help activate our body more healthily.

"In the Kundalini tradition, there are seven distinct energy centres known to exist in the human body, located up and down the spine and also in the brain itself. In a more contemporary scientific understanding, the inner energy vortexes empowering the human organism are understood in terms of the electromagnetic dynamics of subatomic physics. The chakras are in fact a primal expression of the cosmic dance described by subatomic physicists as a spontaneous shifting of matter into energy, energy into matter and matter back into energy again.

"As Einstein clearly posited and ancient yogic masters knew many thousands of years before our bodies are not just material in nature. They are also quite definitely energetic in nature. Science has amassed considerable knowledge concerning this electromagnetic, bio-energetic function of the human body. But scientists are first to admit that they don't really understand the underlying forces that generate life. Scientific instruments can look only so far into the matter-energy range, before reaching their percentage limits.

"Remember, there are 7 Major Chakras, every Major Chakra has 3 Medium Chakras in them and every Medium Chakra has 3 Mini Chakras in it, with the exception of Throat & Solar Plexus Chakras which have 2 Medium Chakras each. So that makes 21 Major and 21 Medium Chakras that a total of 42 Chakras and though every Medium Chakra has 3 Chakras each with the exception of Solar Plexus & Throat Chakras which have 2 Mini Chakras each that's a total of 19 Chakras but, there are 258 Mini Chakras in the body located in various points. An approximate of ± 300 Chakras in all."

"Every Chakra emits an aura which the human body consists of the Inner and the Outer Auras being the main Auras."

THE CROWN CHAKRA

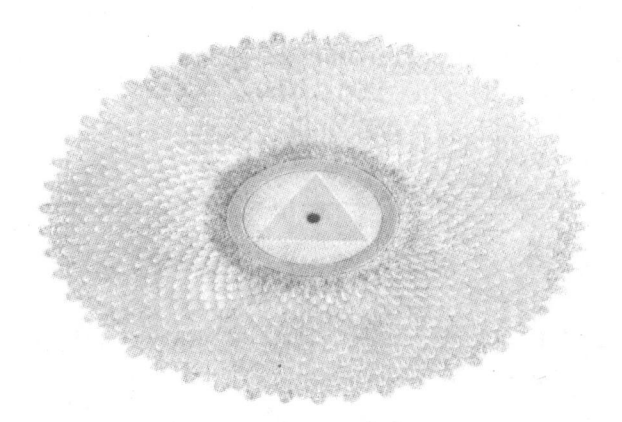

The Crown Chakra is the swirling energy vortex located right in the top of our head and swirling also above the top of our head, where we transcend individual consciousness and tap into infinite consciousness. We come to exist as a separate entity when we are in the seventh-chakra, consciousness. The "ME" evaporates. There is only infinite consciousness, of which we are an integral part."

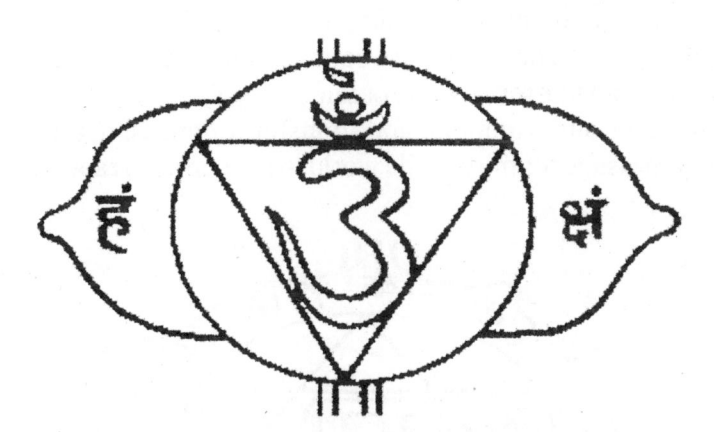

THE THIRD EYE CHAKRA

The first five chakras have been located down below the mind itself. Now, with the sixth chakra, second from the top, we reach the point where we are consciously focusing, the mind is finally looking directly at itself. Whereas the fifth chakra is the chakra of sound, of relatively slow vibrations passing through the medium of air molecules in our planetary atmosphere, the sixth chakra is the chakra of light, of vibratory energy traveling remarkably fast, not needing an atmospheric medium for its transmission.

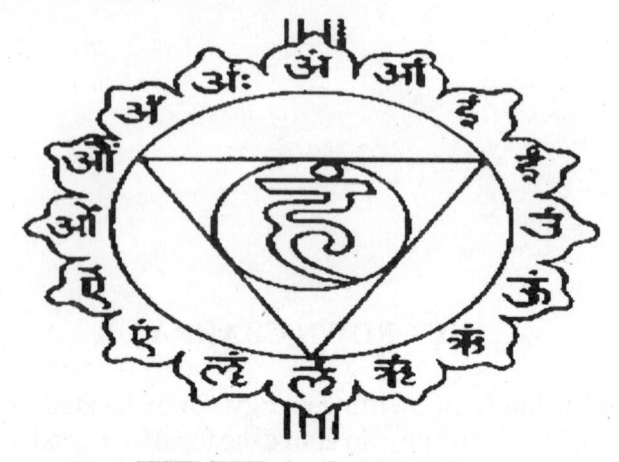

THE THROAT CHAKRA

The throat chakra is the chakra of interpersonal communication. Without it there would be no interchange of ideas from one person to another, and, virtually not human civilization at all. It makes perfect sense for the communication chakra to be in the throat region of the body, since this is where our basic communication tool is located the larynx. Through this remarkable organ we are able to take the outflow of air through our windpipe, and, transform the rushing air into a vibratory message for the outside world to pick up and respond to.

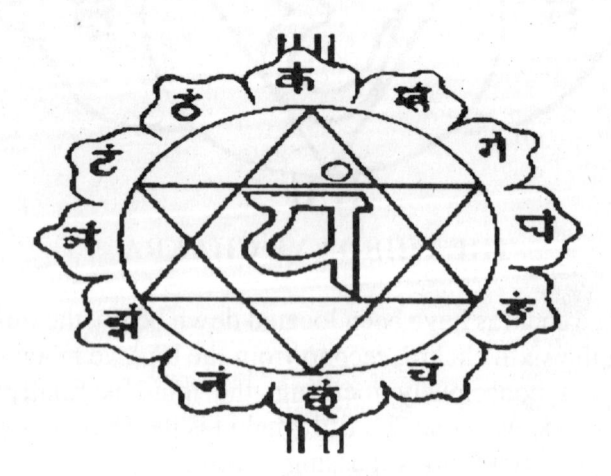

The Heart Chakra

The heart chakra is associated with a magical quality a quality we call love, which ideally serves as the underpinning of all the other chakra qualities of the human energetic system. The heart chakra, in its most basic sense, is the marriage of matter and spirit, of concrete and abstract, of knowledge and wisdom, of earth and heaven. It lies at the centre, and, when balanced with energies from above and below, serves as the true location of the creative force of the universe in the human body.

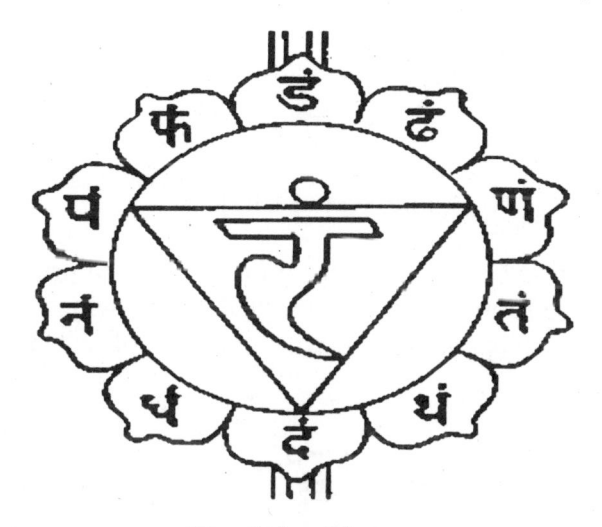

The Solar Plexus

This chakra is beautifully complex energy centre; it deals with personal power, organization capacity, and, the ability to go into action to manifest our ideas in the physical world. This chakra is also linked with the tendency to employ occult powers to manipulate the environment and fellow human being. In a more positive light, this chakras power is used to initiate contact with the spiritual dimensions of life that become more fully developed as we awaken the higher chakras.

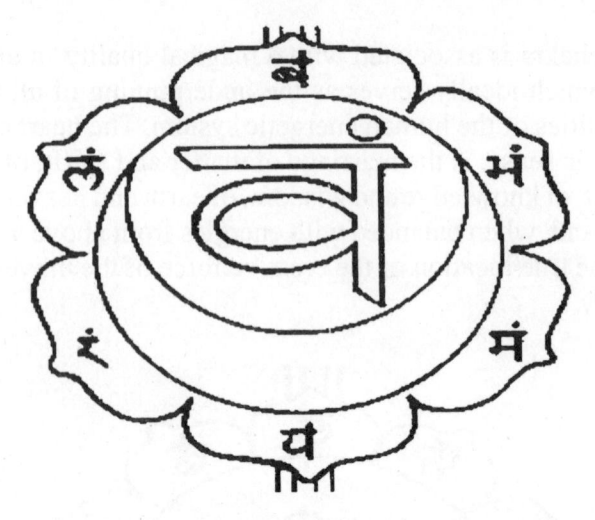

The Sexual Chakra

The key function of the sexual chakra is to manifest primal creative energy into the form of functional sexual energy which the nervous system can then transmute into higher vibrations of spiritual energy.

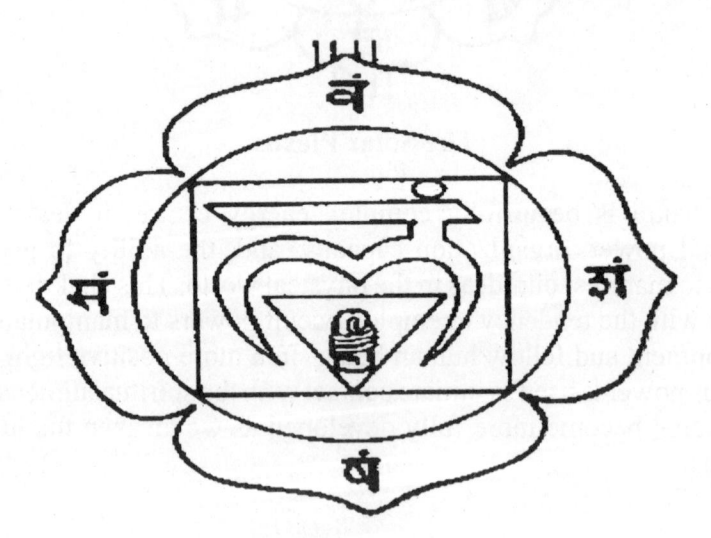

The Root Chakra

The Root chakra is the first chakra from the bottom and the 7th chakra from the top. This chakra is most powerfully related to our contact with the earth, our home planet. They physical nerve bundle at the base of the spine that is associated with the root chakra does look like a massive root system that leaves our spine and runs down both legs like a massive root system down both legs as the sciatic nerve. This is the largest peripheral nerve system in our body. It is as thick as our thumb and it leaves the sacral plexus at the base of our pelvis and spreads like a great root system down each leg, all the way to the tips of our toes and the bottoms of our heels.

Some people consider this root chakra a lowly, unimportant energy centre. Others, especially in recent years, revere it with utmost respect. So, the root chakra, which provides us without connection to mother earth at a most primal level, should be held as equal to the crown chakra at the top of the head.

"Is everything clear?"

There is a nod from every one. Notes are being taken down and some are underlining and putting a question mark on their papers. Questions are coming up, but, when, we have to wait and see.

"Now, we move to Auras"

This is tabulation on chakras:

Name	Position	Colour	Combination
Crown	2" to 3" above head	White, Electric Violet, Golden	Higher Spirituality, Spiritual Life Force, Grace
3rd Eye	Between Brows	Indigo	Inner Sight, Perception, Intuition
Throat	On Throat	Light Blue	Communication, Expression
Heart	On Heart	Light Green	Love
Solar Plexus	3" above navel	Muddy Yellow	Feelings, Emotions, Judgments, Power
Sacral	On Sexual Organ	Bright Orange	Creativity, Assimilation, Elimination, Sexual
Root	Base of Spinal Cord	Dark Red	Physical Survival, Connection with Earth

Name of Chakra	Deity	Divinity	Petals	Mantra	Tattwa
Crown	Paramashiva	Maha Shakti	1000	—	Bliss
3rd Eye	Sambhu	Hakini	2	Om	Light-Mind
Throat	Sadashiva	Shakini	16	Hum	Spirit
Heart	Isa	Kakini	12	Yam	Air
Solar Plexus	Rudra	Lakini	10	Ram	Fire
Sacral	Vishnu	Rakini	6	Vam	Water
Root	Brahma	Dakini	4	Lam	Earth

AURAS : Some Pictures

Chakras

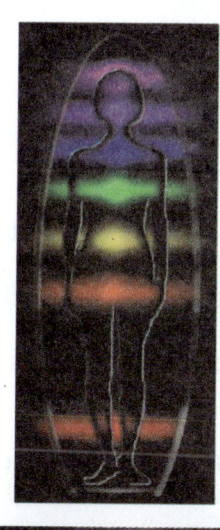

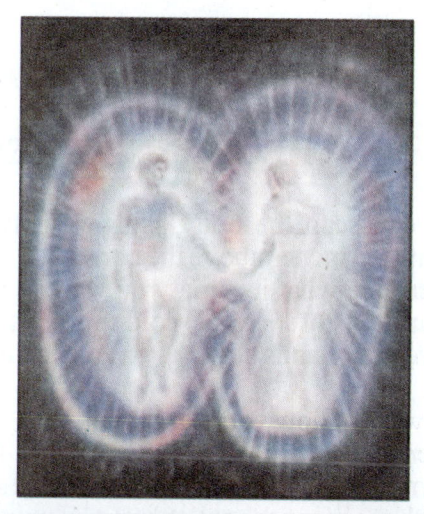

Lovers

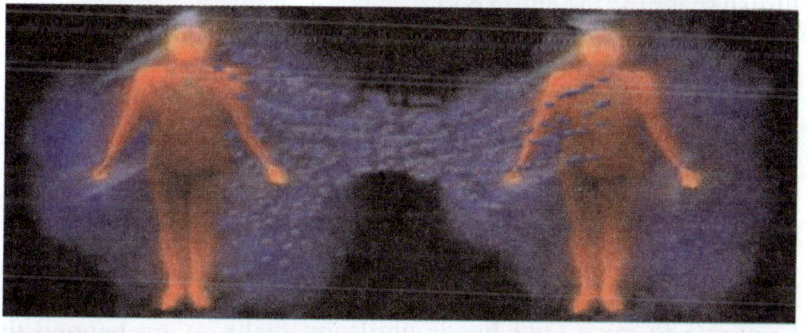

Merging Auras

Aura Movements

Aura Movements

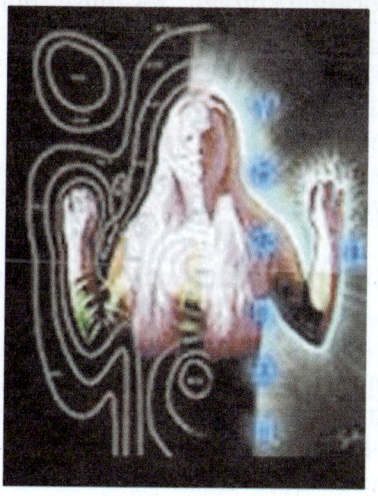

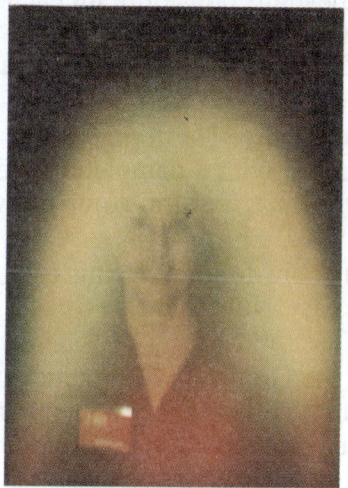

REIKI 1

DAY 1
CHAPTER 10

THE SCANNING TECHNIQUE

- You can scan the body using your two "sensitized" hands held about 1 - 3 inches above the body.
- Determine what it is that you want to respond to.... (a) Stickiness in aura, (2) hot spots, (3) cold spots, etc.
- Move your hands slowly from the top of the head to the soles of the feet.
- Be aware of how your hands feel.
- When they detect anything different (your intended "response") then remember the location(s) of these sensations.
- Finish scanning the entire body.
- When finished, go back to the areas that had sensations, and place your hands on the body....
- Now, slowly raise your hands straight above that area until you feel a sensation; sometimes your hands feel a stickiness (or other sensations) there.
- Hold your hands at that height for about 5 minutes or until you feel a "lightening" of that sensation.
- You can also ask your "Reiki guide/intuition if that area is complete.
- Continue to raise your hands until you feel you are beyond the auric field…in most people, it is about 3 feet.
- Repeat this procedure for each location you felt "response" during scanning.
- Follow up this procedure with a complete "hands-on" treatment.

"From this we learnt that we do not know our Reiki Guide and the procedure with a complete 'hands on treatment' we shall learn this shortly. First, we form groups of two. Please choose partners."

Groups are formed. Being even number of students, pairing up is quite easy. Now, there are 6 paits.

First the Group A will practice on their partners the Group B, then Group B will practice on their partners Group A. After which we will discuss our experiences. But, first let us do the two things-Our Reiki Guide and the hands on treatment technique."

REIKI 1

DAY 1
CHAPTER 11

ON THE ROAD TO SPIRITUALISM

"Supposing this Cosmos is a lift. You get inside the life and enter the 3rd Dimension. When you step out, you immediately enter an immense hall. Everything you have ever imagined is available there. But, everything is in chaos, there are no identification labels, no tags at all. It will take you months to find the things you want.

"You re-enter the lift and go to the 4th Dimension. There is little order here, but, still the items have no tags on them and the lanes are not identified with the type of item in each rack."

"You re-enter the lift and go to the 4th Dimension. There is little order here, but, still the items have no tags on them and the lanes are not identified with the type of item in each rack."

"Now, you go to a higher dimension the 5th Dimension. YES. All lanes are properly identified. All boxes properly labelled. But, a big board at the entry says "Not for taking away.""

"When you start to excavate the thoughts in your mind about your wants/desires/needs, you suddenly find that you have none of these in this 7th dimension.

"Your head bows down. You leave and come back to the 3rd Dimension."

"You do not understand. You are at a loss of words. You re-enter the lift and go to the 6th Dimension. Everything is as in 5th Dimension, the board "Not for taking away" is not there. You feel pleased with yourself. You hand reaches out for a beautiful shirt. But, it passes through the box you understand that is just an aura."

"Immediately, you make a decision. You know the 7th Dimension is the last dimension. You take the lift to this 7th Dimension.

"An Archangel greets you as soon as you step out of the lift. This last immense hall is completely empty.

"You look at the Archangel with questioning eyes. The Archangel smiles. A telepathic message is sent to you. *"Wish and it shall be yours"* *"What do I wish?"* you ask in your mind. The Archangel responds *"Anything in this universe"*

"Now, you have the power to Materialize, to create, the world is yours. The only criteria being, you have to go to the 7th Dimension.

"So!!!! What are you waiting for??? Sit in Meditation and travel upwards to realise your dreams"

The Master smiles – *Message delivered oh esteemed one.*

REIKI 1

DAY 1
CHAPTER 12

SELF-HEALING TECHNIQUE - THE HAND POSITIONS

After the Reiki Master/Teacher gives the attunements to the student, you will feel the warmth of your palms increase.

In a moment we will learn the hand positions and you have just to follow the instructions. After memorizing the hand positions, you will have to give Reiki to yourself as illustrated in the next few pages:

The hand positions are as follows:

1. Eyes - both palms covering both eyes
2. Temples - both palms covering both temples
3. Ears - both palms covering both temples
4. Forehead & Back of the Head - Any way you feel comfortable- one hand on forehead the other on back of the head
5. Both Hands at the Back of the Head - One hand over the other- then at the back of the head
6. Throat Chakra - One hand on Adams apple the other at the back of your neck
7. Thymus & Thyroid Glands - both hands just an inch and a half away from the Adams apple
8. Heart Chakra - Both hands in the center of your breasts
9. Solar Plexus - Both hands on point between the thorax and the navel cord
10. Liver - Both hands on liver
11. Lung Tips - both hands on both the lung tips
12. Pancreas/Spleen - both hands on Pancreas/Spleen
13. Hara - (4 fingers below the navel cord) - both hands on Hara
14. Spermatic Cords (Gents) Ovaries (Ladies)
15. Thigh (Right) & Thigh (Left)
16. Knees (Right) & Knees (Left)
17. Calf-Muscles (Right)) & Calf Muscles
18. Ankles & Sole of Foot (Left)

REIKI 1

DAY 1
CHAPTER 12

SELF-HEALING TECHNIQUE - THE HAND POSITIONS

After the Reiki Master/Teacher gives the attunements to the student, you will feel the warmth of your palms increase.

In a moment we will learn the hand positions and you have just to follow the instructions. After memorizing the hand positions, you will have to give Reiki to yourself as illustrated in the next few pages:

The hand positions are as follows:

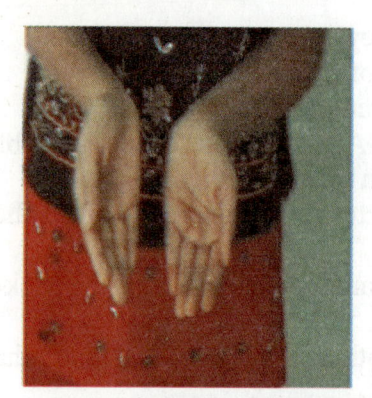

Cup your hands as above

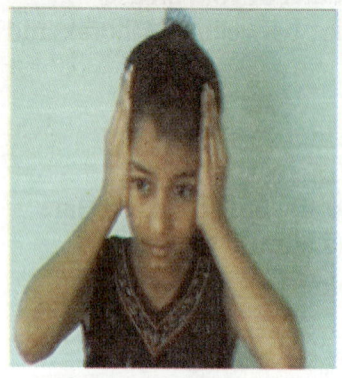

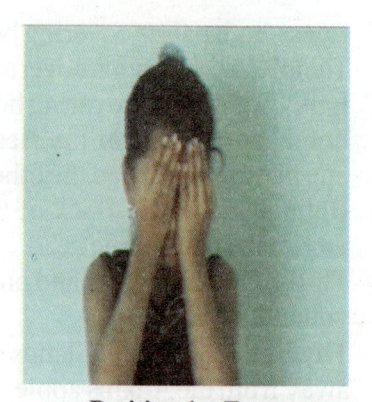

Position 1 – Eyes

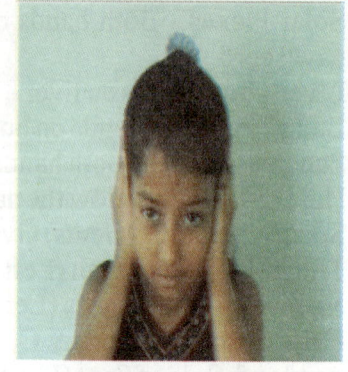

Position 2 – Temples

Position 3 – Ears

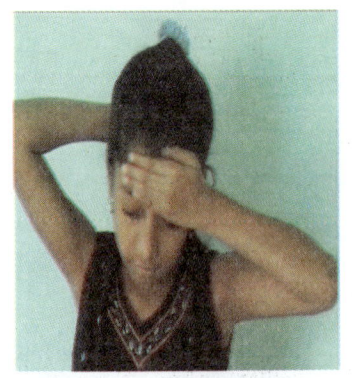

Position 4 – Front & back of head

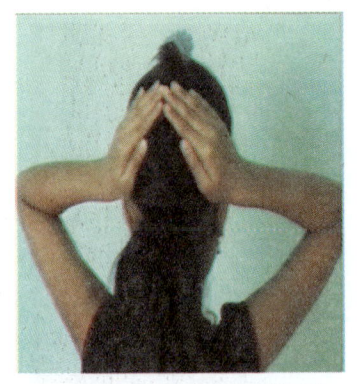

Position 5 – Back of Head

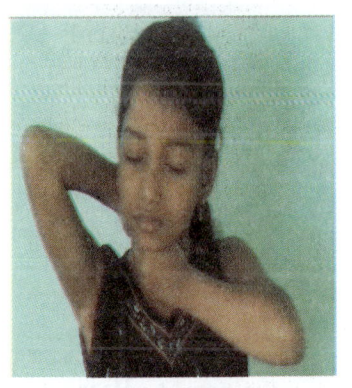

Position 6 – Front & back of Throat

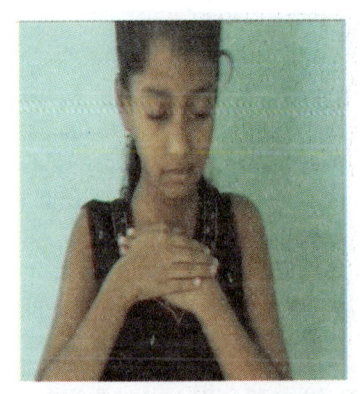

Position 7 – Thymus & Thyroid

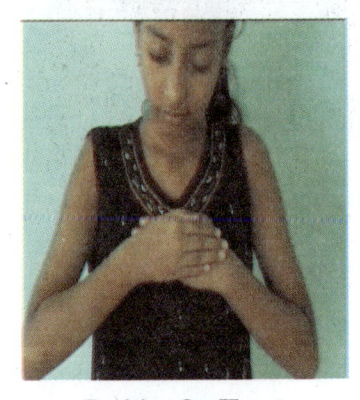

Position 8 – Heart

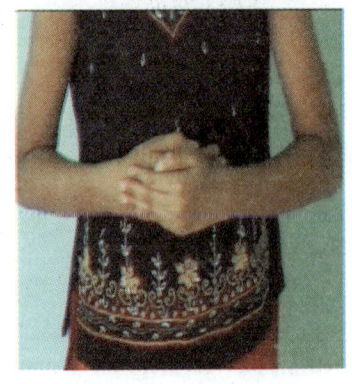

Position 9 – Solar Plexus

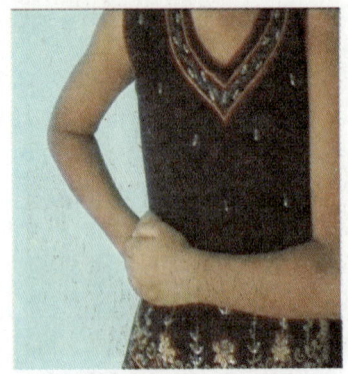

Positi on 10 – Liver

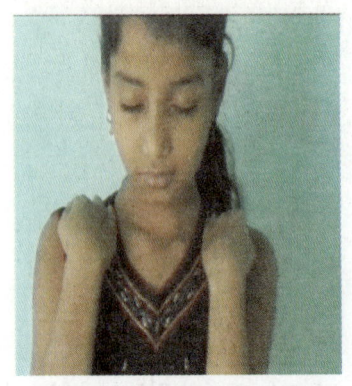

Position 11 – Shoulder Tips

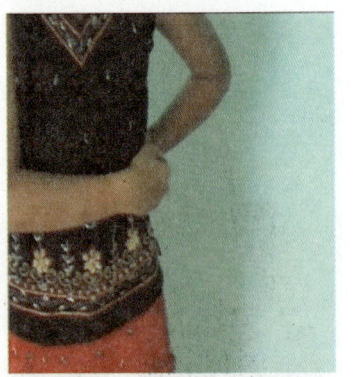

Position 12 – Pancreas & Spleen

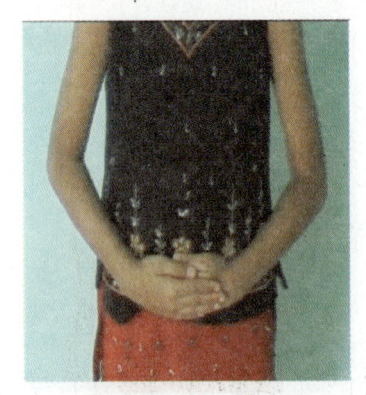

Position 13 – Hara

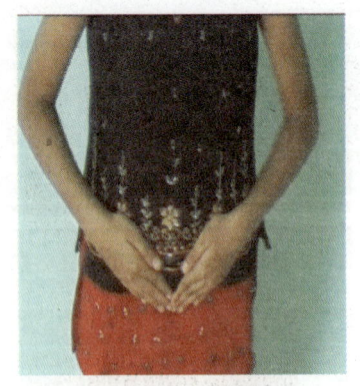

Position 14 – Ovaries for Women
Spermatic Cords for Men

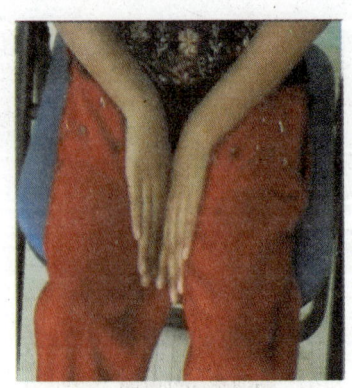

Position 15 – Thighs

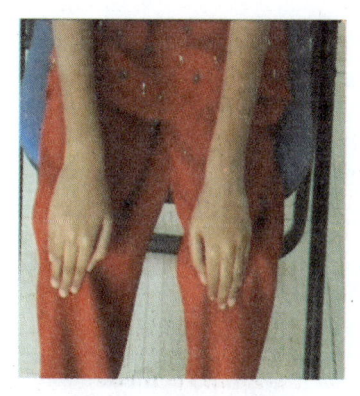

Position 16 – Knees

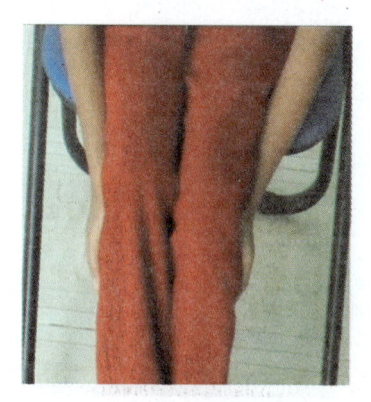

Position 17 – Calves

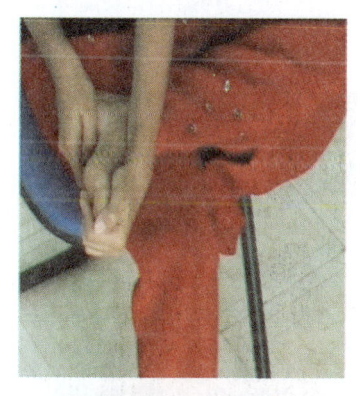

Position 18 – Foot left

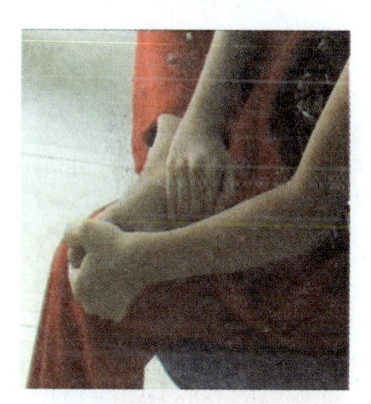

Position 19 – Foot Right

ILLUSTRATIONS – BACK SIDE OF THE BODY – 7 POSITIONS

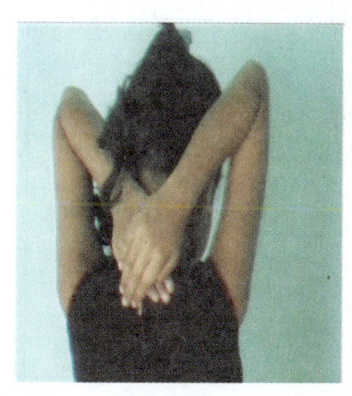

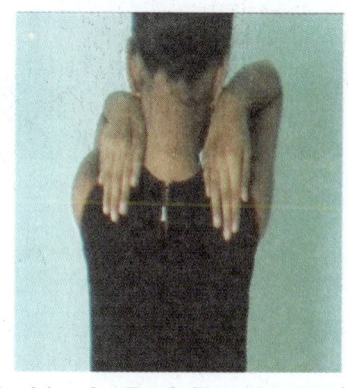

Position 1 – Back Thymus Thyroid

Position 2 – Back Shoulder Blades

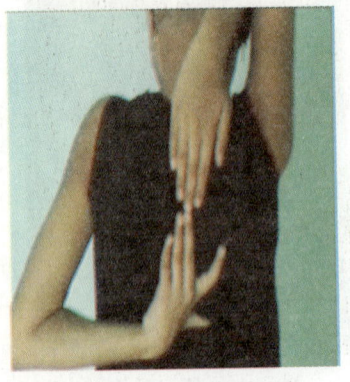

Position 3 – Back Heart

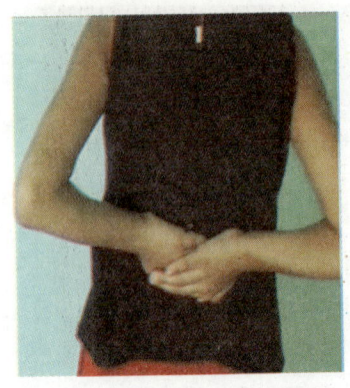

Position 4 – Back Solar Plexus

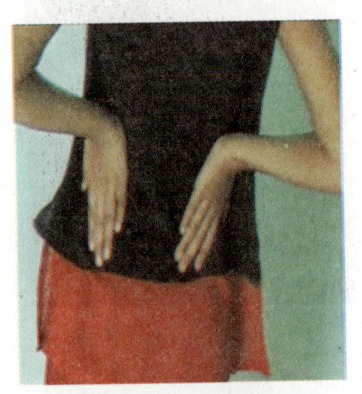

Position 5 – Kidneys

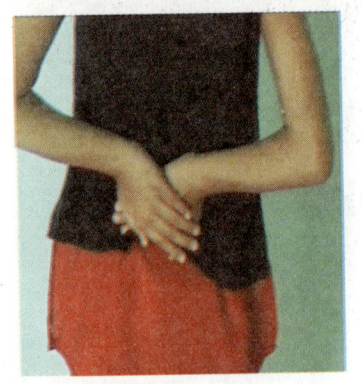

Position 6 – Hara

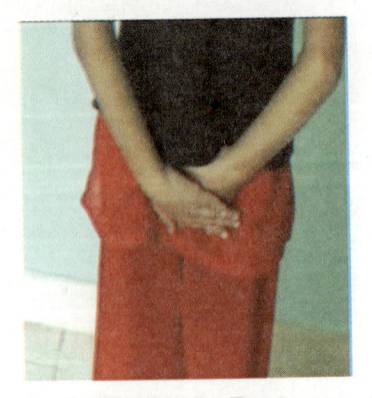

Position 7 – Root

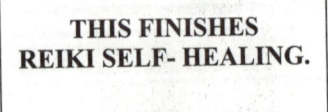

**THIS FINISHES
REIKI SELF- HEALING.**

REIKI 1

DAY 1
CHAPTER 13

DO'S & DON'TS ABOUT REIKI

DO'S
- Wash hands before and after giving Reiki - to stop the flow of energy
- Have a conversation with the patient, ask him why the healing is required
- Convince him to come for at least 3 to 4 days
- Patient should wear loose clothing, empty his/her pockets, take off their rings & watches, belts and all/any metals.

DONT'S
- Reiki Patients should not cross their legs while taking Reiki Energy
- Every point covered must be for a minimum of 3 minutes - though the Reiki channel may or may not feel the energy passing through the palms.
- Do not make any diagnosis

POINTERS:
- DAY 1, the patient may be withdrawn, knot knowing where the hands will be moving
- DAY 2, he/she will accept the movements of the hands and probably fall asleep as relaxed
- DAY 3, he/she may wait for some experience
- DAY 4, will experience REIKI ENERGY

PLEASE TAKE CARE TO:
- Keep a jug or glass of drinking water handy
- Keep tissue paper handy
- Explain to the patient that we are just Reiki Channels and the patient will be drawing as much energy as it required by his body.
- Always start Reiki with the Head Position
- Spirals after the front body - from RH to RL & from LH to LL
- Chakra balancing on the back
- Caressing, also known as the evening of AURAS.

REIKI 1

DAY 1
CHAPTER 14

WHAT IF YOU COME ACROSS COLD AREAS?

When you become a Reiki Channel and start using Reiki to treat your friends and relatives, you will notice at times, that some of the parts where Reiki is being given are cold. (I.e. you will not feel any warmth in your palms nor you will feel that the patient is absorbing any energy) So what do you do???

1. Cup you hands and scrape the area where you feel cold, visualize there is a burning cauldron kept next to you, after scraping the area, throw the scraped waste into the burning cauldron. Repeat thrice.

OR

2. Visualize pulling out strands of hair from the cold areas, one by one, then tie a knot to the strands of hair and throw it into the universe.

ELSE

3. Visualize there is a bucket of salt water kept next to you. Do any of the above, and throw it into the bucket with the salt water.

By adopting any one of the above techniques, you will feel the cold areas are becoming warmer.

Continue with the Reiki session.

REIKI 1

DAY 1
CHAPTER 15

VISUAL MEDITIONAL EXERCISE
THE GLASS TECHNIQUE

(As explained in Silva Mind Control Classes)

The Glass of Water technique is a mental technique that can be used for problem solving and goal achievement. This technique is mostly taught in the Silva Mind Control Classes.

As being a graduate in the Silva Mind Control, I have personally studied and practiced this technique and can promise you one thing - IT WORKS.

Whenever, you come across a hurdle, a problem, that cannot be crossed or solved, do the following:

"At night just before retiring fill a glass of water and take it to the bed. When you are about to go off to sleep, cup the glass in your palms and look for 30 seconds into the water in the glass and repeat 'I know I have (state the problem)' - then close your eyes, look towards the ceiling of the room, and repeat mentally 'This is all I need to do to find the solution to the problem I have in my life'"

Drink away half the water.

The other half can be covered and kept aside.

In the morning when you wake up, before going into your routine chores, taking the half filled glass in your hands, repeat your problem mentally, and say "Today, I will find the solution to my hurdle/problem" Drink away the balance half of the water.

What will happen is this:

Anytime during the day that follows, a message may be conveyed to you by anyone, either you're favorite TV soap opera; conversation with a friend, a taught from yonder; a remark passed by a friend. Anything. Just be on the look out.

Just in case, nothing follows, repeat the exercise again the next night - it works like magic.

Good luck.

REIKI 1

DAY 1
CHAPTER 16

COLOURS FOR HEALTH

RED:
Unlimited energy, used in cases of blood diseases

ORANGE:
Digestion & assimilation of oxygen through the respiration system, particularly in cases of asthma and all diseases involving the lungs and chest area.

YELLOW:
For purification and also for diseases such as diabetes and those affecting the intestines and bowels.

GREEN:
Revitalizing the nervous & circulatory system and also the heart.

BLUE:
Tranquility and peace, also, used for destruction of all forms of infections.

INDIGO:
Treatment of all illnesses and diseases affecting the area of the head, the eyes, the ears and the nose, mostly for treatment of mental and emotional disorders.

VIOLET:
Regeneration of the nervous system, for curing insomnia, mental disorders resulting from brain damage, physical illness and injury affecting the brain itself and diseases and injuries to the eyes.

WHITE:
Unlimited energy for the treatment of all diseases and injuries. Treats the body and mind as a whole and is especially useful when a specific diagnosis of the individual's sickness for injury has not or cannot be

made.

BLUE-GREEN:
For reduction of pain.

COLOURS TO BE AVOIDED IN CERTAIN SITUATIONS:

RED:
If emotionally upset, hysterical or extremely overtired. The vital energies present in this colour can overload an individual with too much energy and make sought-after tranquility more difficult to achieve.

GRAY:
If emotionally depressed. In situations where an individual has allowed himself/herself to give in to negativism concerning health or a situation of life, Grey should be totally avoided.

BLUE:
By individuals who find themselves depleted in physical or mental energies. When the physical, emotional or mental energy levels are low, blue in clothing or surrounds should be avoided.

REIKI 1

DAY 1
CHAPTER 17

THE 'OM' MEDITATION

Each day, just before the session of Reiki comes to an end, a short simple meditation of 30 seconds to one minute is to be carried out.

1. All students stand up and form a close circle
2. All hands are to be put on the shoulders standing on the right and left side of you.
3. Close your eyes.
4. Chant "OM" (Actual sound AHHIIIIHHH......UHHHHHHHH......OHHHHHH to end in a vibratory MMMMMMMMMM)
5. The chant is to be repeated thrice.

This is the OM Meditation.

REIKI 1

DAY 1
CHAPTER 18

SUMMARY

What we have learnt so far can be divided into 3 parts.

Part One is the Visual Meditation Exercises, which help us in treating this WORLD and the people living in it with the White Light Meditation. The Lily Pond teaches us to negate our negativities and clean ourselves of all diseases. The Glass Technique teaches us to get the answers from yonder. Be Alert, this technique say.

Part two are the Art of Living by Dr. Goenka where we can learn to harness our bitterest enemy - OUR ANGER and of course with this goes the OM Meditation to subside our ego, our desires and calm our nerves.

The Colors teach us many things, what we wear, what we eat, what friends we have, speak a lot about ourselves. Make it a prime factor in your lives and see the difference it makes in your life.

Reiki - The Chakras - We have learnt to give Reiki through the Chakras, via, Self-Healing technique. The Chakras harmonize our body. The most important thing to remember is the color of each chakra. Mix the color and it will bring a major disaster in your life.

<u>NO QUESTIONS ARE BEING ASKED AT THIS STAGE, BUT, TOMORROW AFTER COMPLETING THE REIKI 1 SESSION, WE HAVE SHALL SOME QUESTIONS, WHICH I AM SURE YOU WILL BE ABLE TO ANSWER SPONTANEOUSLY.</u>

REIKI 1

DAY 2
CHAPTER 1

REIKI 'A' ON 'B' & 'B' ON 'A'

When you start giving Reiki to a person, you have to repeat the following:

For attitude and for gratitude -

" I thank myself for being here
I thank Reiki for being here
I thank (insert the name of the person being treated) for being here"

Visualize a cloud above your head. Visualize the cloud emitting white light over you. Feel the white light falling on the top of your head and traveling from your Crown Chakra to your 3rd Eye Chakra, from your 3rd Eye Chakra to your Throat Chakra and from your Throat Chakra to your heart Chakra. Visualize the white light bouncing off from your heart chakra to your shoulders and from there flowing into your arms. Visualize the white light traveling from your arms into your palms. Visualize the white light emitting from your palms when you start giving Reiki.

Start Reiki.

REIKI THE FRONT SIDE POSITIONS

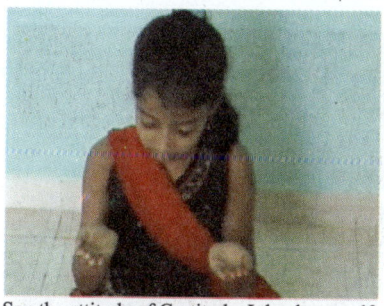

Say the attitude of Gratitude. I thank my self for being here. I thank Reiki for being here I thank (patient's name) for being here - start

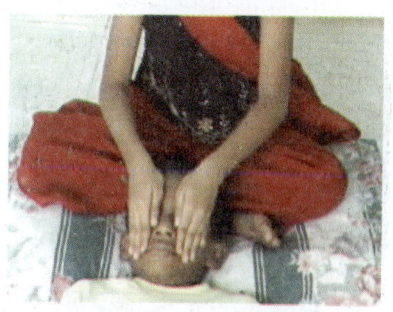

Position 1 – The Eyes

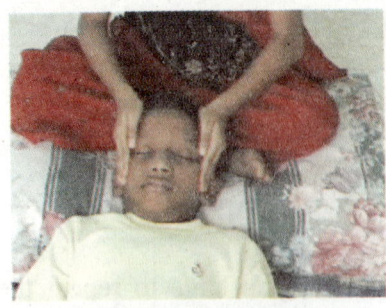

Position 2 – Temples

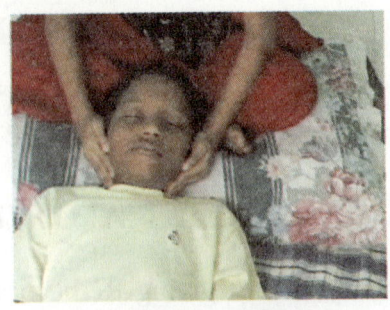

Position 3 – Ears

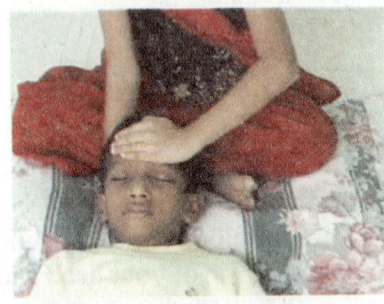

Position 4 – Front & back Of neck

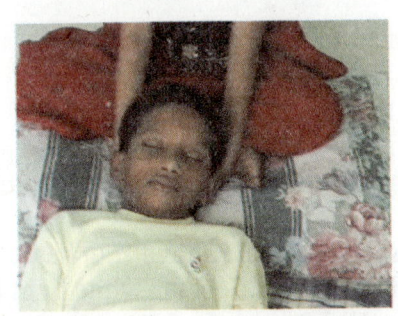

Position 5 – Back of Head

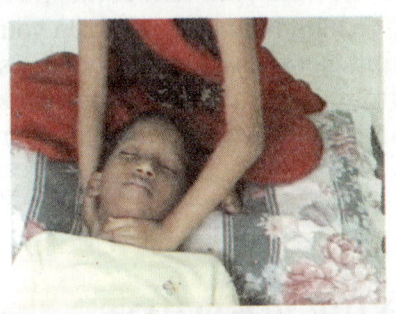

Position 6 – Front & back of the neck

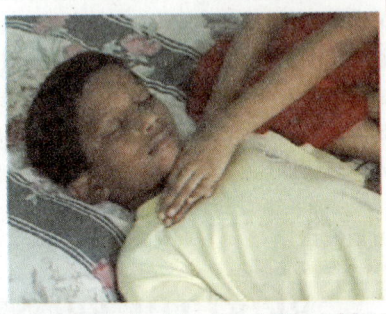

Position 7 – Thymus/ Thyroid

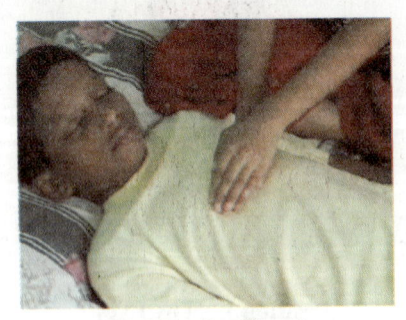

Position 8 – Heart

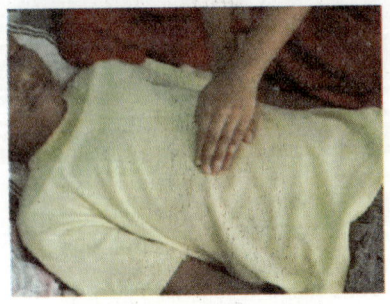

Position 9 – Solar Plexus 3" above navel cord

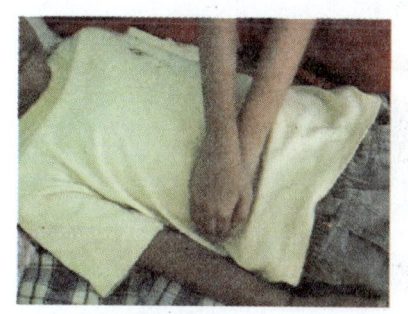

Position 10 – Liver

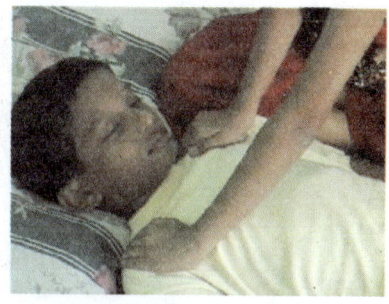

Position 11 – Shoulders

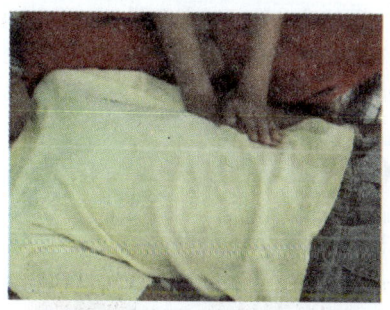

Position 12 – Spleen/Pancreas

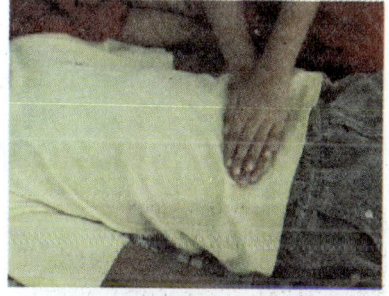

Position 13 – Hara
(3" below navel cord)

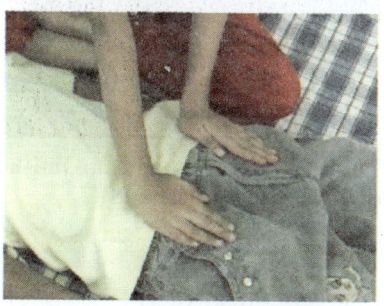

Position 14 – Spermatical Cords / Overies

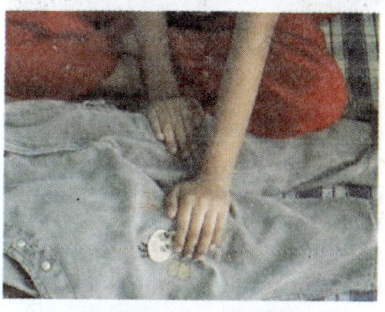

Position 15 – Thighs

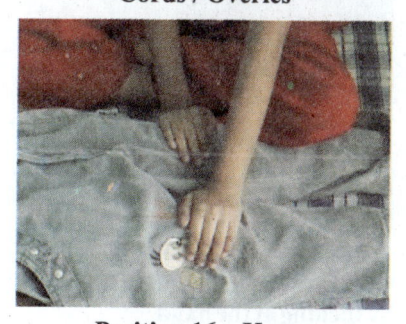

Position 16 – Knees

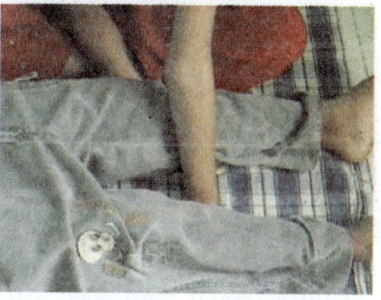

Position 17 – Calves

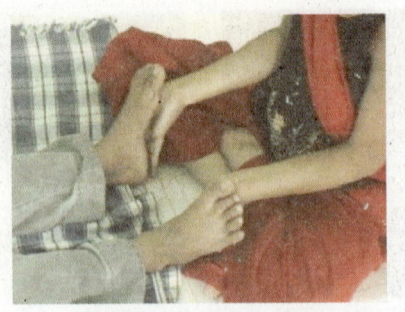

Position 18 & 19 – Feet

This finishes Reiki on the front side of the body. Before the patient is told to change his position and sleep on his stomach, we have to do the spriralling technique which is as follows:

THE SPIRALLING TECHNIQUE

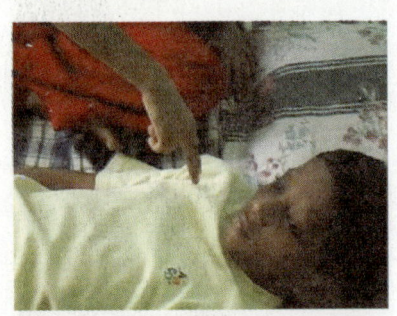

The Index & Middle pointed, rest of the fingers folded in the palms. Point the two fingers on the Right Shoulders, do small anti-clockwise motions, and slowly move towards

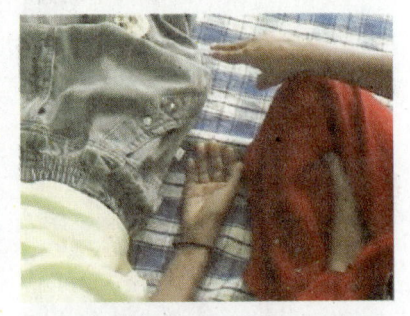

The tip of the right hand and finish off by flicking at the hand

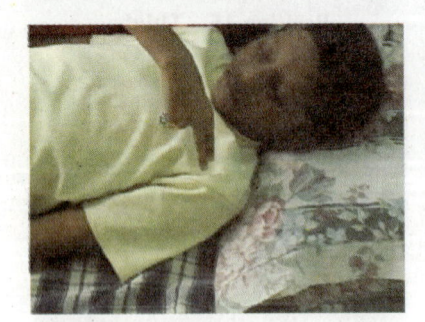

Same way as before on the left shoulder, small anti-clockwise motions and move towards

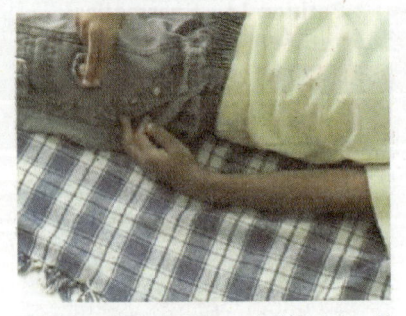

The tip of the left hand & finish off by flicking at the hand

54

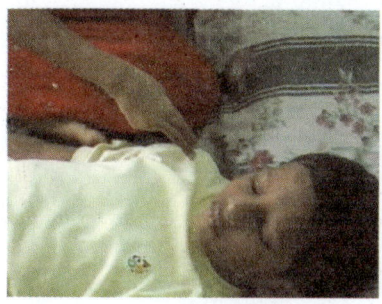

Same way to be continued, this time from right shoulder

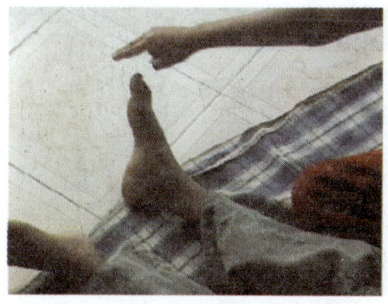

Finish off by flicking at the feet.

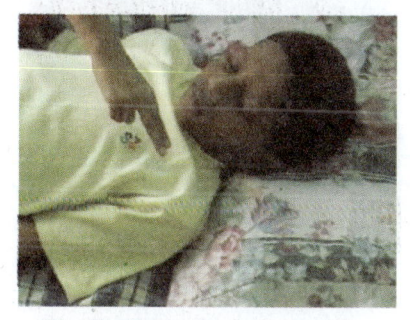

Finally, from the left shoulder

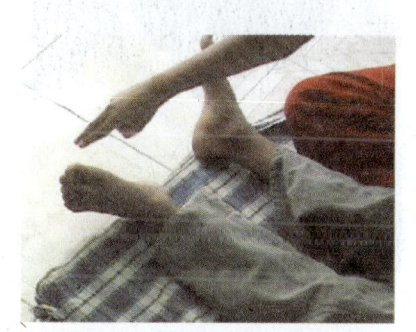

Finish off by flicking at the feet.

The patient is now requested to shift position and sleep on his stomach.

The back positions start now.

THE BACK POSITIONS

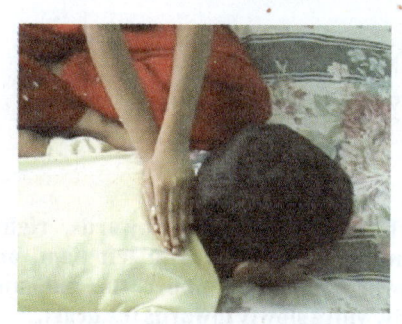

Position 1 – Back Thymus/Thyroid

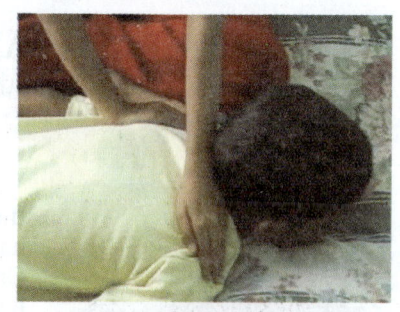

Position 2 – Back Shoulders

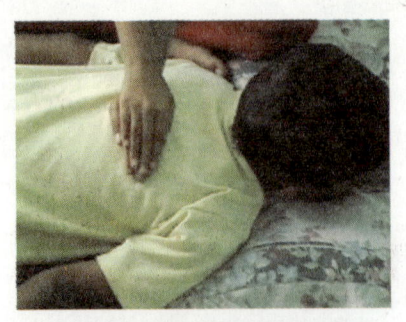

Position 3 – Back Heard

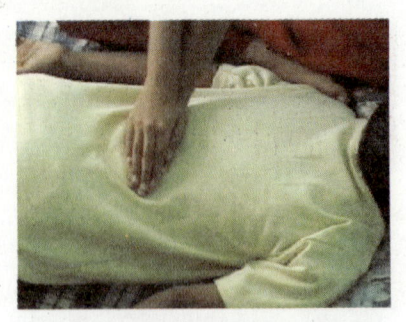

Position 4 – Back Solar Plexus

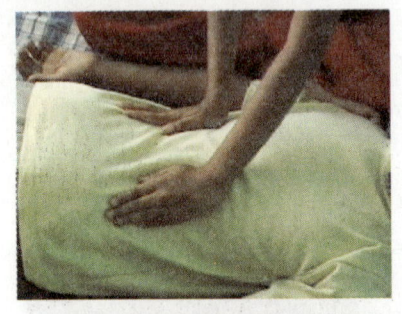

Position 5 – Back Kidneys

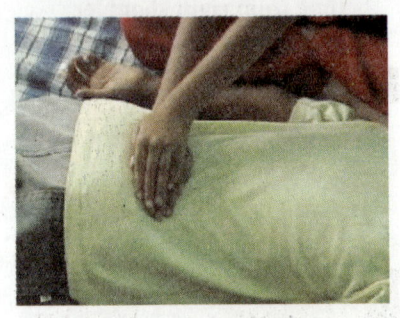

Position 6 – Back Hara

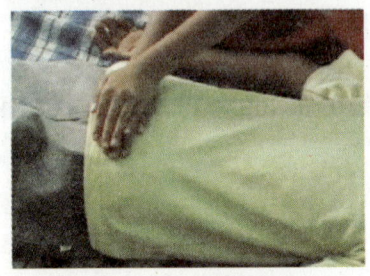

Position 7 – Back Root

This finishes Reiki on the back part.

THE CHAKRA BALANCING TECHNIQUE
Now, we have to do the Chakra Balancing.

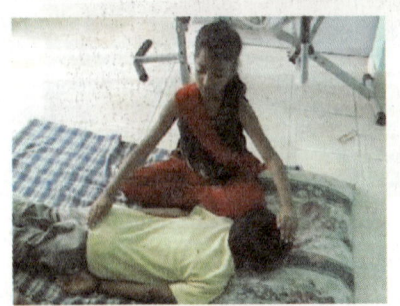

Both palms facing downwards, right hand on Root Chakra & left hand on Crown Chakra 3" above the patients body. Move slowly towards the heart.

Both hands meet at the heart thumb to thumb. Wait for 5 seconds. Move to next position.

Both palms facing downward, move to position 2 - right hand on Hara & left hand on 3rd Eye Chakra 3" above the patients body. Move slowly towards the heart.

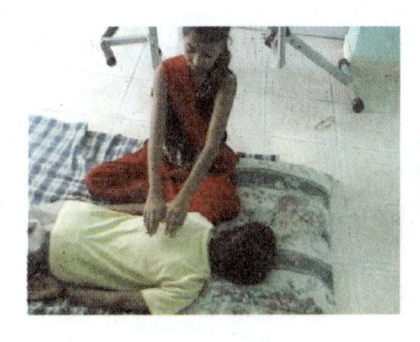

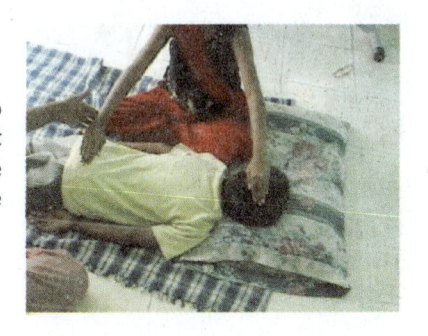

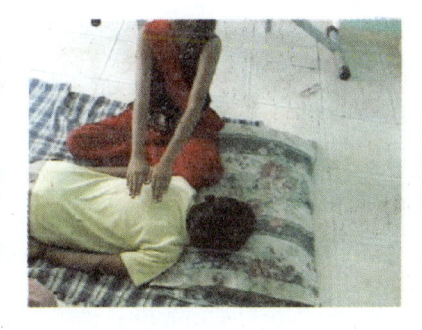

Both hands meet at the heart thumb to thumb. Wait for 5 seconds. Move to next position.

Both palms facing downward, move to position 3 - right hand on Solar Plexus and left hand on Throat Chakra 3" above the patients body. Move slowly towards the heart.

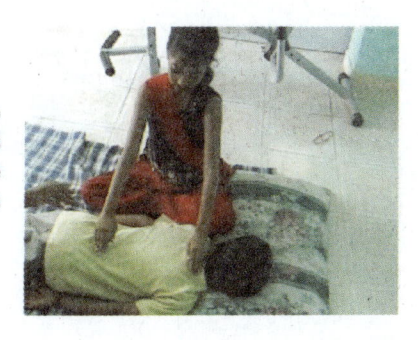

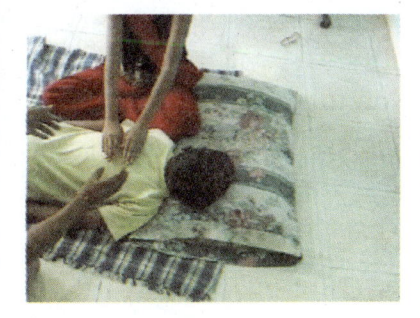

Both hands meet at the heart thumb to thumb. Wait for 5 seconds. Move to next position.

Both palms facing downward, move to position 4 - right hand on Heart Chakra & left hand on Solar Plexus 3" above the patients body. Move slowly towards the heart.

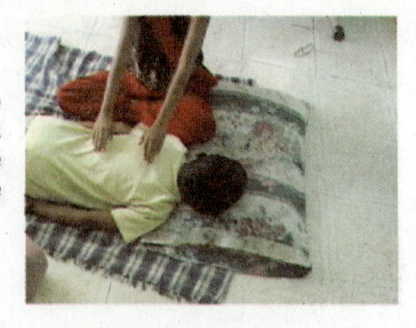

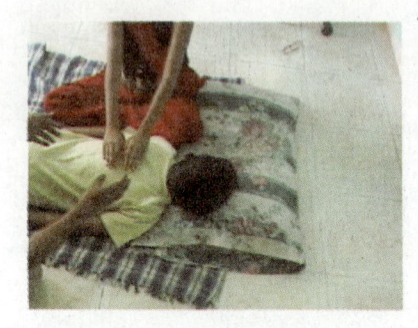

Both hands meet at the heart thumb to thumb. Wait for 5 seconds. Move to next position.

Move back to Solar Plexus & Heart position Position No.4

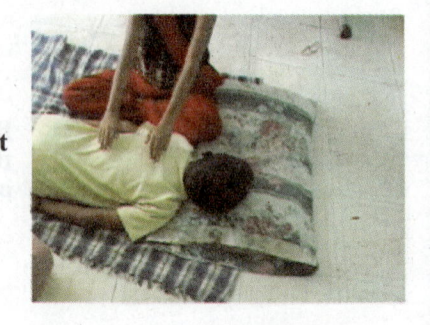

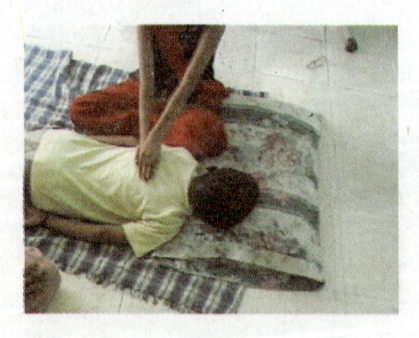

Both hands meet at Heart Chakra, right hand on the heart & left hand on top of the right hand. Press slightly.

This completes the chakra balancing. Now to complete we have to do the stroking as follows:

58

THE STROKING TECHNIQUE

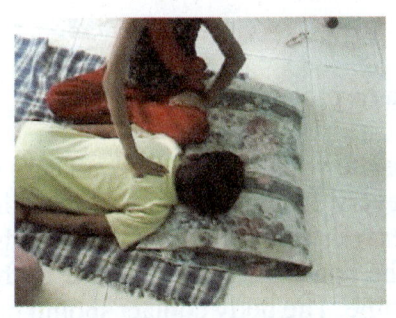

3 fingers from top of the neck   draw your hands to the root in one quick motion. Do it thrice.

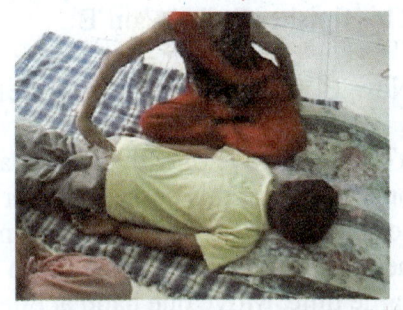

There is still one more technique before Reiki 'A' on 'B' is complete. Caressing.

THE CARESSING TECHNIQUE

Theory

Keep your left palm on the back of your right hand. Place this on the head of the patient and do as follows:

Remember, not to lose contact with the body throughout the complete process.

1. Covering head caress slowly and move towards the right shoulder and down toward the patient's hand. Move backwards towards the head in the same way.
2. Now, repeat the above process towards the left shoulder and down toward the patient's hand. Move backwards towards the head in the same way.
3. Now, move towards the right shoulder and in a straight line downwards towards the right knees and feet. Same way move backwards towards the head.
4. Now, move towards the right shoulder and in a straight line downwards towards the left knees and feet. Same way move backwards towards the head.

5. Caress from head to Heart Chakra. Press slightly.

This finishes Reiki 'A' on 'B'

Now 'B' will do Reiki on 'A' in the same process as explained.

You can always play the Reiki cassette while giving Reiki. There is only music in this cassette. After every 3 minutes you will hear the sound of a BELL. Proceed to the next position as soon as you hear the bell. Remember one thing, both the hands should not move at the same time. Move one hand at one time. The body contact should not be left at any time.

When you come to the feet position, do the 3 minutes Reiki individually on each foot.

This exercise was given by my Guru:

- Sit in meditation
- Go to Alpha Meditation.
- Breathe in deeply, more deeply up to your *Root Chakra.*
- See red colour surrounding this Chakra.
- The Root Chakra is expanding East to West and North to South.
- Now, look at the Crown Chakra.
- Breathe in light Golden Colour.
- See light Golden Colour surrounding this Chakra.
- The Crown Chakra is expanding East to West and North to South.
- Now, look at the Heart Chakra.
- Breathe in light Light Green Colour.
- See the light Green Colour surrounding this Chakra.
- The Heart Chakra is expanding East to West and North to South.
- Now, look at the 3rd Eye Chakra.
- Breathe in Indigo Colour.
- See the Indigo Colour surrounding this Chakra.
- The 3rd Eye Chakra is expanding East to West and North to South.
- Now, look at the Sacral Chakra.
- Breathe in bright Orange Colour.
- See the bright orange Colour surrounding this Chakra.
- The Sacral Chakra is expanding East to West and North to South.
- Now, look at the Throat Chakra.

- Breathe in light Blue Colour.
- See the light Blue Colour surrounding this Chakra.
- The Throat Chakra is expanding East to West and North to South.
- Now, look at the Solar Plexus Chakra.
- Breathe in Muddy Yellow Colour.
- See the Muddy Yellow Colour surrounding this Chakra.
- The Solar Plexus Chakra is expanding East to West and North to South.
- Visualize now a pillar has been formed from your root chakra to your crown chakra.
- Sit in this pillar devoid of any thoughts.
- Sit as long as you feel or till your eyes open automatically.

REIKI 1

DAY 2
CHAPTER 2

SERIOUS CASES

As a Reiki Channel at times you will be called to treat cases, which are more of a serious nature.

What do you do?

Accept these cases. Advise the next of kin of this people, tell them what Reiki is, the nature of Reiki is and how the treatment is affected.

Advise them that as the person is in a serious condition, no guarantees on his life can be given. Be honest, but do not be negative. Tell the next of kin of the patient, that you are not to be held responsible if anything-untoward things happen. In most of the European countries, you may be taken to the court.

Reiki is not a mumbo-jumbo practice. It is Universal Energy. Reiki passes through every problematic area into the body and heals the person by itself. It is out of our hands to control this energy.

For the first few days, there may be no results. Then from the 5th day onwards the patient may show some positive signs. Most probably from 12th to 14th day or so, the toxins start leaving the body; hence the patient may have a relapse.

Do not get worried, continue with the Reiki Sessions, probably do MARATHON REIKI on the patient.

REIKI 1

DAY 2
CHAPTER 3

The Reiki Marathon

Reiki is not limited to healing; it is a spiritual discipline which calls more of our Spirit essence into the physical body, thus connecting together more of our "wholeness" with our multi-dimensional selves and with the Godhead.

This means we have more energy to work with in this plane of existence, and therefore, less wear and tear on the body. When we do not have much Spirit residing in our body, we get out of balance, and begin to put strain/stress on the systems, which keep us in good health and balance. This can lead to imbalances that if not corrected, will have to be dealt with by medications, or even surgery. And if not corrected, we may meet with death because of system failures.

Reiki practitioners have been taught the only task necessary to 'charge our batteries' is to place our hands on specific areas of our body and the energy will act as a slow-charge to the organs that keep our systems in good working order. But most practitioners have also been taught it only requires one hour-per-day to return our depleted systems to full energy and vibrant health. For some, this may be true, but for many others, one hour-per-day has not proven to be sufficient. Every body requires varying amounts of energy before "enough" has been stored to begin the re-balancing of all bodily systems.

We teach practitioners that a minimum of three days of treatments is necessary before the body can begin to draw upon the 'charged' energy and start to eliminate/change the conditions, that have limited the body's flow of energy. More often than not, a person who has had a long standing or chronic condition(s) will need much more than three consecutive days of Reiki treatments. Of course this is difficult because of time constraints and busy schedules of both the practitioner and the recipient alike. When time just does not allow for three or more consecutive treatments, some practitioners have learned to give whatever they can; some Reiki is better than none.

This is true to a point, but if a recipient hopes and desires to regain health and vitality, then some Reiki may only be a 'teaser' and may not be enough to show any change of conditions. What can be done? How can a recipient receive enough Reiki energy to sufficiently 'quick-start' the re-balancing (purification) of a dis-eased organ or system?

The Reiki Marathon may be the answer. We know the word 'marathon' means "An event or activity which requires prolonged effort or endurance." The Reiki marathon, then, is a specific chosen period of treatment time performed by multiple practitioners. Here is one way this may work.

Talk to all the Reiki practitioners you know in the area. Ask your Reiki friends to contact their Reiki friends for a soon-to-be-held Reiki Marathon. Schedule a convenient date for the recipient when s/he will be available for the whole day, or the greatest part of it. Schedule a minimum of one practitioner to do hands-on treatment every hour throughout the day. Try to cover every hour without break.

Group therapy in these types of cases works wonders.

Reiki may be given to the patient for one and a half hour by each group of 4 to 6 people continuously for 6 to 9 hours daily.

Do not worry about results, as Reiki is a positive and an intelligent energy, think positive and hope for the best that the results will be positive.

REIKI 1

DAY 2
CHAPTER 4

GROUP HEALING

Group healing is ideal for Chronic diseases like: Cancer, Aids, Asthma, Arthritis, Diabetes, Chronic Rheumatism, Lumbago, fever, blood related problems, etc.

A group may consist of 4 to 6 Reiki channels treating the patient at one time.

Usually the most experienced person may take over the charge of the Reiki channels, but anyone who takes over the head position is considered to be the person in-charge for that particular session.

We have studied that there are 19 positions on the front side of the body, if the thighs, the knees and the calves are taken as 1 position each.

If the thighs, knees and the calves are taken separately than there are 22 positions on the front side of the body and 7 positions on the back side.

The person taking over the head position usually works out a chart.

Supposing you are the head person, how would you work out a chart?

First, including you how many other Reiki Channels are there?

Supposing 6.

How many total Reiki Positions are there in the front side.... Total 19 (taking the thighs, knees & calves as one position each).

As you are taking the head position, and there are 5 positions in that area, (Eyes, Temples, Ears, Forehead, Back of Head) first we have to minus these 5 positions from the total of 19 positions. Balance positions left are 14 only.

Because the Root Chakra is equally important to the Crown Chakra, we leave one person to do the feet, as these are counted to be the extensions ruled by the Root Chakra. That is 2 positions. This will again leave a balance of 12 positions to be divided amongst the 4 people.

We have already placed 2 people,

1 - at the head
1 - at the feet

The other 4 will be seated as follows:

Person No. 1: On the Right hand side - will take The Throat Chakra, The Lung Tips, Thymus & Thyroid Glands, the Heart Chakra.

Person No. 2: On the Left hand side - will take the Solar Plexus, The Liver, The Pancreas/Spleen and the Hara

Person No.3: On the Right Side - will take the Spermatic Cords/Ovaries (Depending on sex of the person), Thigh - Right, Thigh - Left

Person No.4: On the Left Side - will be Knee right, Knee left, Calf - Right & Calf - Left.

All Reiki Channels raise their hands, palms facing upwards and say the "Attitude of Gratitude"

"For attitude and for gratitude
I thank (state you name here) for being here
I thank Reiki for being here
I thank (state the name of the patient) for being here.

The Reiki Music cassette is played. On sound of the bell the hand positions are changed. All the Reiki channels know their positions before hand. As some of the Reiki channels have less positions and some more, the ones having less positions, will stop at the last position and continue giving Reiki to that part till the others complete their positions.

The person on the head position will do the Spirals for the front side.

For the backside there are only 7 positions,

1. The person on the head position can take the Shoulders & Thymus/Thyroid Glands.
2. The second person - the heart Chakra
3. The third person - the Solar Plexus
4. The fourth person - the Kidneys
5. The fifth person - the Hara
6. The last person - the base of the spine (Root Chakra).

Again, the person in the head position will complete the session with the Chakra Balancing, the Stroking and the Caressing.

This completes the chapter on Group Healing.

REIKI 1

DAY 2
CHAPTER 5

VISUAL MEDITATIONAL EXERCISE
YOUR FAVOURITE PLACE
&/OR
YOUR SANCTUARY

In every human life, there comes a day when you are frustrated, disillusioned, finding that you are in the lowest ebb of your life, you are frantic …

And in this state you want one thing … TO GET AWAY FROM IT ALL.

To have a place, where you are alone with yourself. You do not want any outside force to ever see you again. You wish to be just alone, in a SECRET PLACE only which you know of.

But, is there such a place???

Let's approach this from a different angle. But, before we do so, let me ask you a question. Okay?

- Which is the fastest mode of transport?

Think before you can answer.

I will answer this one for you: The fastest mode of transportation is your **"IMAGINATION"**.

In the beginning of the book, I have mentioned that the inner self is much more bigger than the outside world. Comparatively, the outside world is smaller than the inside world.

So, why look to hide on the outside. Why do we not take our imagination, our visualisation on the inside?

We create our own hiding spot, in the mountains, on any planet in the Solar System, under the earth, above the earth, anywhere. But, this world of ours will be inside us. Nobody can find us there.

We know how we expose ourselves to the world, clean, pious, caring for others, but we also know what is inside us, don't we?

So, let's make a hiding place inside us. The ideas of the snow clad mountains, forests, ponds, rivers, forests, can be taken from the outside, but this world will be our world in the inside of us.

- Do your breathing exercise, breathe in to the count of 4, hold your breath to the count of 4, breathe out to the count of 4.
- Continue with deep intakes of breath, till you feel a little dizzy or till you feel relaxed.
- Visualize yourself in your favorite place of relaxation.
- Visualize you are taking a stroll in your favorite place of relaxation, where no other human being, animal or bird is allowed to enter without your permission.
- As you are strolling, visualize that there is a cloud following you.
- Look up at the cloud. This cloud looks great.
- Visualize that as you are looking at the cloud, the cloudbursts open and a force of white light descends on you.
- Feel as if millions of bulbs have been lighted up.
- Visualize the colours of the rainbow, the violet, indigo, blue, green, yellow, orange, red, lilac, white.
- Feel the tingling sensations in your body.
- Feel as if you are being carried away on the wings of a big bird.
- You are feeling light, very light.
  All you worry, negativities, fears have been washed away by the light from the cloud.
- Mentally bow down and whisper "I thank you lord for the mercy shown to me, for giving me the power to fight back and rise up, thank you, thank you, thank you my lord"
- Look up at the cloud again, it has vanished.
- Keep strolling in your favorite place of relaxation.
- You do feel relaxed - isn't it??

Come back to the room as and when you feel you are ready to fight back and rise again.

REIKI 1

DAY 2
CHAPTER 6

WHEN NOT TO GIVE REIKI

I recollect a case, where a person has a major problem with the calves (legs). He was overweight and was a chain smoker. He approached me for treatment. It is my habit, to talk at length with the person requesting for Reiki. While counseling him, I came to know that this was a chronic problem he had.

He could never sit on a sofa or a chair for more than a few minutes. Every day when he came home after the office hours, he would lie down on his back and keep his feet on the center table for at least 30 minutes. He had tried every form of cure, but to no avail.

I started with the 21 days Reiki course and during the days that followed I felt his full body was cold. Sometimes, energy just wouldn't pass from my hands. He was not accepting energy. I was surprised. Then, on the 9th day, I visualised the valves of heart were clogged. I saw him gasping for breath. Then I saw him turn blue/greenish in colour. I started sweating. When I opened my eyes, he was smiling at me.

I stopped attending him. On the phone I advised him that something would happen. What, I had an idea but did not want to tell him about it at that time.

On the 12th day, he called me and said, "Do you know where I am sitting?" I was perplexed. He answered "On the Sofa" he paused, and then continued "Thank you very much for curing me. I have fired my family doctor. He could not cure me for the last 8 years, and, you have shown me results in just 9 days"

During the conversation I requested him to visit a cardiologist with me, I let out my fears on him and told him what I had visualised. He laughed.

Anyway, we went to the cardiologist. The Cardiologist took an x-ray and we found out his heart was enlarged. But, I knew, this was not what I had seen. We attended another clinic, where the doctor showed me his valves on a TV Screen. They were perfectly healthy.

But, the fear in me would not go.

On the 14th Day, since I had started giving Reiki to him, and the 5th Day, since I had stopped giving Reiki to him, as he was not accepting the energy, I got a call from him, he just said "I am sweating a lot and also I am feeling choked up" intuitively, I knew it was a heart-attack. I advised his friend who was with him, to call for an ambulance and rush him to a hospital.

I disconnected the line, called my friend's wife, advised her to rush to the hospital, and, took a cab myself to the hospital. My friend was brought on a stretcher and taken to the ICU. Within the next 25 minutes, he was pronounced dead.

The reason, I gave you the above incident is, anytime while treating a patient; you may come across a similar incident.

That is, while giving Reiki, you may feel that there is no energy passing through your hands, you may not feel any sensations, which you as a Reiki Channel are supposed to feel.

When the Soul is preparing to leave the body, it will not accept any energy from any source.

During these types of cases just excuse yourself and **DO NOT GIVE REIKI TO THAT PERSON.**

REIKI 1

DAY 2
CHAPTER 7

VISUAL MEDITATION EXERCISE
YOUR COUNSELLORS

Time will come, when you will seek advise from people around you, asking questions:

- This person I am treating is suffering from throat cancer (optional), I am nervous, what if while giving Reiki, I catch the disease?? Can you tell me what to do??
- I have been treating Mrs. XYZ for more than a month, but she doesn't seem to be responding, what shall I do?
- Mr. ABC coughs a lot when I give Reiki to him, I am nervous, what if I catch the virus and fall sick myself?
- Reiki is taking it's own course, it takes a lot of time to heal, how can I heal the person faster?

Questions, questions & questions.

But, there are answers to every question. Isn't it??

Sometimes, we tend to ask questions to people who do not know the ABC of what we are doing. So, are they qualified to answer??

Sometimes, we tend to ask questions to qualified people, but again who do not know the language of Meditation healing techniques, they scoff at these techniques. Are they qualified to answer our questions?

So, who is qualified? Who will not scoff at you? Who is the person who will appreciate the pains you are taking to heal people known and unknown to you? Who will listen to you patiently; discuss your problems with you. Who is the person in your mind whom you trust, whom you respect??

Select such 2 persons - One Male & One Female.

Now, as you have selected these 2 persons, we will do one more exercise.

- Visualize yourself in your favorite place of relaxation.
- Visualize you sitting under the shade of a tree and remembering these persons we were talking about.
- Utter one of the person's names on your lips. Visualize that person. See him standing in front of you.
- In this place, you do not need to speak, telepathy works here.
- Gave way to your thoughts. Request this person, whom you cherish, respect, love, to become your Councilor. Request him, you need his advise on matters pertaining to the sickness of the people, their depressions, their mental, spiritual, physical problems, which at times you fail to understand.
- Look out for the first thought. If it is "YES", he is chosen to be your Councilor. If "NO" look out for another person.
- Repeat the same with the other person - request her to be your Councilor
- Look out for the first thought. If it is "YES", she is chosen to be your Councilor. If "NO" look out for another person.
- Relax - come back to the room whenever you feel like.

These Councilors will always help you with your medical cases when you come across hurdles, which you may seem difficult to cross.

REIKI 1

DAY 2
CHAPTER 8

VISUAL MEDITATION EXERCISE
YOUR LABORATORY

PLEASE NOTE THAT THIS IS NOT A REIKI EXERCISE.

We now have, our Secret place of relaxation.

We also have, our own Councilors.

What happens when Reiki fails to cure?

When going through the Reiki course, I remember, my Reiki teacher's wife was having a problem, which Reiki could not cure. I was requested to ease the pain of this sweet and loving lady. I did what was necessary and she was excused from taking those 8/10 odd tablets she takes as her usual dosage.

What about Manjusha, she is also a Reiki Master. Still she could not cure her mother's illness of Frozen Shoulders.

Maybe, both my Reiki Teacher and Manjusha are at fault, they talk about Reiki, my Teacher teaches Reiki, but do they have the patience?

If they do, then Reiki is a failure, but, if it does not, then this is not the system, which is wrong, it is the people.

Maybe they are lacking in Love & Compassion for their fellow beings???

There are too many maybes. But, the choice is yours to decide.

To make the ART OF HEALING COMPLETE, I shall be teaching you 3 more arts during this Reiki Course, which shall make your healings complete.

You can treat anyone of any disease with 100% results.

Coming back to this Chapter, we may need to give treatments to the people in Absentia. By absentia, I mean, when they are not physically present.

How do we do that?

Simple.

We make a UNIQUE LABORATORY, where we have all the treatment facilities, which a human mind can conceive.

First, we do the normal breathing exercise.

Then, when we are feeling relaxed, we go to our favorite place of relaxation.

From here, we go to someplace else and make a Laboratory.

THE EXERCISE

- Visualize yourself erecting a Laboratory with your mental thoughts.
- Visualize yourself inside the main hall of this laboratory
- Mentally call in your Councilors
- Visualize your Councilors are in your presence.
- Mentally discuss with them what you need in this laboratory.
- Visualize yourself erecting a big screen.
- Mentally repeat the following "By the power given to me by my Supreme Self, I instill the power in this screen, to show the places of defect in the human body when the person is placed behind it"
- Visualize a computer in front of you.
- Mentally repeat the following "By the power given to me by my Supreme self, I load this CPU with the most successful programmers on the healing techniques ever conceived by a human mind"

Mentally converse with your Councilors requesting them to be present in this Laboratory for 24 hours a day for the rest of their lives, inventing cures for diseases, which the world has failed to

cure.
- Visualize them smile and affirm to your request.
- Mentally, seek their permission to leave.
- Come back to the room whenever you feel you are ready to do so.

For this exercise, you have to be careful to do the following:

- Always wish your Councilors individually whenever you enter or leave the Laboratory.
- Never think negatively when in the Laboratory
- There is a cure for every disease in this Laboratory.
- The Councilors are always present in the Laboratory to listen and to advise you.
- Your entry to the Laboratory is always first, then if you wish you can call your patient
- Discuss the patient with the Councilors first then call the patient to this Laboratory.
- Do not converse with the patient in the laboratory. Just treat him/her.
- In serious cases, the mental image can be left under a white light till further notice.
- Operations can be performed to the best of your and the Councilors knowledge.
- While treating the heart, always remember to stop the clock. After the heart is treated, you can start the clock again.
- Remember; do not touch the patient's heart, till the clock is visualized in stopped position.
- The more clear the mental pictures, the more fast the treatments/results will be.

REIKI 1

DAY 2
CHAPTER 9

MEDITATION

"David" I called out to one of my students during the Reiki Classes

"Yes" he tuned in

"Can you tell me - What is Meditation?"

"It is an art where you sit down doing nothing, and, the results are, you achieve everything"

BRAVO. I could not have explained better.

If you want the doors to be thrown open to you to plunge yourself into the world of light, the world of love, the world of truth, PLUNGE yourself into MEDITATION. Meditation will lead you to the ultimate goal of your existence and self-realization.

The next natural question asked would be: How do we meditate?

We meditate in 4 different ways, similar to the wheels of a car.

1. The first wheel is to focus on our inner self.
2. The second wheel is the use of a Mantra, a word or a syllable that assists in concentration
3. The third is an asana or the sitting posture that supports the body and stimulates the nervous system.
4. The fourth wheel is the breath, balancing the twin process of inhalation and exhalation.

Let's divert ourselves a little. We talk about our relaxation - about sleep. When we feel sleep taking over us, we shy away from our wife, our children, food, T.V. ... Everything that we believe gives us comfort. During our sleep, the weariness washes away and when we wake up - we feel completely relaxed.

We experience this everyday. If we ponder on this subject, we will realise, all the external activities we engage ourselves during the day, exhaust us. But, the internal activity (sleep) rejuvenates us. So, eating, drinking, partying, T.V. are not the permanent pleasures that will bring us peace.

When we sleep we are peaceful. During the day the mind turns outwards. However, in the sleep state, the mind takes some rest in the self, and, it is this, which removes our fatigue. Absorbed in this little bliss of sleep, we forget the pains of the waking state. If we were to go just beyond sleep and enter into the state of Meditation, we would be able to drink the nectar of love and happiness, which lies in the heart.

This nectar is what we are looking for in all activities of the outer world. What we are really seeking is the supreme truth, and, through Meditation we can experience this truth vibrating in the form of sublime happiness in the heart.

The truth is that you are divine. It is only the wrong understanding that keeps you small. You think yourself as only a body. You think you are in a certain physical structure, with hands, feet, legs, eyes, ears, mouth…

You differentiate yourself by sex - a man, a woman, by class - by race - by nationality. You identify yourself with your thoughts, your talents, your positive and your negative actions. But this is not what you are.

Within you is a being that knows all the actions of the body and the mind, and, remains untouched by all of them. The body is a temple; the being inside you is the keeper of the temple.

The one, who tends to the temple, has to be different from the temple. For example, you will say "My body" similar to "My Wife" "My children" "My Mother".

Your mother is different from you - hence my Mother
Your children have to be different from you - hence "My Children"
Your wife has to be different from you - hence "My Wife"
Your body has to be different from you - hence "My body"

Who is this keeper of your temple - your body who observes the activities of your waking hours? At night when you sleep, this keeper remains awake and reports to you the dreams you have had in the night. Who is this keeper???

The one who lives in the temple - you body, but who is apart from the body is YOUR REAL SELF. That self is beyond the body, beyond the mind, beyond distinctions of name, colour, sex, nationality. It is the Pure "I", the Original "I" consciousness that has been with us since we came into this world.

What we have done is that we have superimposed different notions on to that "I" awareness. This "I" is not only pure consciousness but is also a form of Bliss. It is the ABSOLUTE. That I - IS GOD, and we meditate to know that directly. As we see it more and more, we become more transformed.

Many techniques are being taught in this world and in the age. But, the oldest art is the art of Meditation. Because, we can see our Inner Self directly when we are in Mediation. That which lives in the heart, cannot be found in the books. It cannot be found in any religion and neither can it be found in any religious books.

Remember, "All books are written by a brain, yes, the brain can make any number of books, but no book can make a brain" Better throw out the books and MEDITATE.

Meditation is universal. It does not belong to any cult or sect. It does not belong to the East or West, or to any religion. Meditation is every ones property just like sleep is every ones property, it belongs to Humanity.

Every one meditates. Doctors, Cooks, Teachers, Painters, Mothers and everyone else.

Any type of concentration on any particular field is known as Meditation, though this meditation is external.

What we have to do is to meditate internally. What does meditation do?

- It rids us of disease and makes us more skillful at everything we do.
- Understanding of Inner and outer things becomes steadily deeper.
- Stills the mind which constantly wanders
- We travel to different inner worlds and have innumerable inner experiences.
- Relieves us of our sufferings
- Establishes us forever in the state of supreme peace.
  Makes us aware of our own true nature.

The physical "I" constantly keeps on changing. From I am a child to I am an adult, I am a brother, I am a son, I am a husband, I am a father, I am a grandfather, I am a clerk, I am a supervisor, I am an officer, I am a manager - I keeps of traveling through different phases all the time.

Meditation is concentration - concentration should be:

- On a particular object in order to still and focus the mind
- One can concentrate on the heart
- On the open space between the eyebrows - 3rd eye chakra
- On any being who has risen above passion and attachment.
- Wherever the mind finds satisfaction.

The best being the inner self. Why not? Don't we need to know our inner self first? Don't we need to experience our self? Remember the bible "What you seek - you get"

Seek thy inner self - and it shall be thine.

When you sit for meditation, do not worry about thoughts evading your privacy. Do not try to erase the thoughts in the mind. Accept them. These thoughts are nothing but consciousness itself.

Let the mind wander as much as it wants to; do not try to subdue it. Witness the thoughts that arise in you. Be whatever thoughts coming to you, just be aware of them. This is but a play of your consciousness. You are also a play of your own consciousness. Hence, the thoughts are nothing but you.

You need a thorn to take out a thorn from your body. Another way to meditate is to put a thought into your mind to avoid the other thoughts from entering your conscious/sub-conscious level. The thought that you are going to use is a "MANTRA"

Either the Mantra will be a one-word syllable like:

"OM"
"AING"
"REEM"
"JEEM"

Or a sentence. Or any positive affirmation can also be treated as a Mantra:

"IF GOD BE FOR ME, WHO CAN BE AGAINST ME?"
"DAY BY DAY IN EVERY WAY I AM BECOMING BETTER & BETTER & BETTER"

Mantra is but a thought, which redeems and protects the one who contemplates it. Mantra is the heartbeat of Meditation. The greatest of all techniques. Mantra is self-vibration, self-speech, and when we immerse ourselves into the Mantra; it leads us to the place of the self.

Mantra repetition should be with reverence during meditation, it begins to work within. This energizes us and awakens our inner energy, our own Power.

What should be our physical posture when we sit in the Mantra Meditation?

There are four postures in which Meditation can be done.

1. The Lotus posture (In yoga this is known as Padmasan)
2. The half lotus posture (In yoga this is known as Siddhasan)
3. The easy posture (In yoga this is known as Sukhasan)
4. The lying down position (In yoga this is known as Shavasan)

The most important of the above is the Lotus position. Because by sitting in this position for a period of 1½ hours, purifies the 72,000 nerves and inner subtle channels. Moreover, the mind will begin to turn inward and Meditation will happen on its own.

BREATHING should be natural and spontaneous. We must not try to disturb the natural rhythm of the breath. The mind and the breath work in conjunction with each other. So let the rhythm of the breathing be natural. As you repeat the mantra, the breath will go in and out in time with the rhythm of the mantra and will become steady by itself.

Meditation on the self is very easy. All that we really need are love and interest. As we meditate more and more, the inner power awakens and begins to unfold.

The inner universe is much more greater than the outer universe, it is so vast that the entire outer cosmos can be kept in just one corner of it. Everything is contained within it, and that is why, in Meditation, the seers were able to discover all the secrets of the universe.

Within us are infinite miracles, infinite wonders. As we go deeper into meditation, we will come to understand the reality of all the different inner worlds we ready about in the scriptures. Within these inner spaces, nectarean music resounds. Within us are such delicious nectars that nothing in this world can compare with them in sweetness. We should meditate systematically and with great persistence and go deeper and deeper within the body. In this way, Meditation will be a gradual unfolding of our inner being.

Along the way there will be many experiences. But, the true state is beyond them. As we go deeper into meditation, we reach a place where we see nothing and hear nothing. Here there is nothing but bliss. This is the place of the self, and, true meditation is to become immersed in that!!

REIKI 1

DAY 2
CHAPTER 10

REIKI WHAT WE HAVE LEARNT SO FAR

We have traveled a long way. From knowing nothing to knowing something - is achieving a lot. Whatever knowledge we gain, will certainly improve our status, our being, ourselves.

What are the important things we have learnt so far?

1. The white light meditation to make this world a better place to leave in.
2. The Meaning and the history of REIKI.
3. The 5 Principles of Reiki.
4. How to control the devil in you - your ANGER - by a discourse by Dr. Goenka in The Art of Living.
5. The Chakras.
6. The Reiki Positions.
7. The Colours for health and their affect on our daily lives.
8. How to give a complete session of Reiki.
9. Group Healing.
10. Apart from Reiki, we have made our own place of relaxation; we have our own councilors and our own laboratory, which we shall use to treat people by the Mind Control & T.V. - Pic methods.
11. We had a very good discourse on Meditation and the art of Meditation
12. Most important is that we have also learnt the art of visual meditation, which gives us peace of mind and builds us up to become better humans.

REIKI 1

DAY 2
CHAPTER 11

QUESTIONS - TIME FOR EXAMINATION

You have worked wonders with yourself. You have been working hard to reach this far. How do you feel at this time and hour? Do you feel satisfied internally? Do you want to know if you are successful? If yes, please answer the following questions:

1. What is Reiki?

2. Why do Reiki Master/Teachers always have the White Light Meditation included in their seminars?

3. What are the 5 principals of Reiki?

4. Why did Dr. Usui Mikao adopt the 5 principles of Reiki?

5. How many positions are there on the front side of the body and how many on the back side of the body, please mention their names also.

6. What is Reiki Alliance & Who started the Reiki Alliance?

7. What would you do when you come across cold areas while giving Reiki?

8. What is group healing?

9. Give a chart of 5 people giving a group healing to a patient. State briefly how the positions will be divided amongst each person on the front side of the body and on the backside of the body.

10. Did you try to do any Visual Meditation Exercises? If yes, which one. What was the outcome of it? What did you feel? How did you feel after completing the exercise?

11. Did you do the attunements? Who did the attunements for you? What was your experience during day 1? Also, what was your experience during day 2?

12. Do you feel you palms are getting warmer than usual? If yes, then what do you think the reason is?

REIKI 2

DAY 1
CHAPTER 1

LET'S DISCUSS YOUR SELF-HEALING/REIKI EXPERIENCE

Welcome back to the advance level of Reiki 2

For those of you who are new to this Seminar on Reiki 2, I would like to introduce myself. My name is Mohan. I will be your Reiki Master/Teacher during these 2½ days seminar.

Before we proceed further, I would like to congratulate you all present for successfully completing the Reiki 1 Course.

The question is - Did you complete the 21 days self-treatment?

If the answer is 'Yes' you may stay back.

For those who have not done the "21 days" self-treatment - please leave this room.

What did you feel during the last '21 days' of giving Reiki to yourself?

How do you feel now?

Do you feel you are ready for the Reiki 2?

I can see the smiles on some of your faces. You look calmer, more peaceful with yourself. Good.

Keep up giving Reiki to yourself - Not only will your body become healthy, your mental powers will increase and so will your attitude towards life. To put it in a nutshell -

YOU WILL BE A BETTER PERSON.

Let's discuss - why we need to do the REIKI 2 Course?

REIKI 2

DAY 1
CHAPTER 2

WHY 2nd DEGREE - A DISCUSSION

The ones who are remaining here presumably have completed the 21 days of self-cleansing. By self-cleansing I mean, all of you must have gone through giving Reiki to yourselves for a period of 21 days.

Some of you may have given Reiki to other people also. How many of you have given Reiki to others?

All?

Good. Could you diagnose the ailments while giving Reiki? Where you accurate in your diagnosis?

How did you feel by becoming a Reiki Channel?

Of course, you must have felt nice; otherwise you wouldn't be here, isn't it?

I am sure some of you must have felt handicapped. Do not be alarmed. I do not use the word handicapped practically; I use the word in phraseology. I will be clearer.

I am sure some of you must have felt inadequate. Some of you must have been approached by family members/friends/acquaintances to treat people who are not physically present, in these circumstances, I am sure you must have felt insufficient.

Do not worry. The reason for doing Reiki 2 is simple.

We learn Reiki in a wider way. By the time this seminar ends, you will be self-sufficient to treat any case, be it physically or in absentia. You will learn to treat all types of diseases. You will also learn to give short form of Reiki. You will become adept at the absentee healing techniques using the tools of Reiki, Mind Control, Colours, and

Crystals. You will also be doing more Visual Meditations exercises, which are serious in nature.

To learn Reiki 1 - was a pleasure. To learn Reiki 2 - will be a pleasure cum business for you. You remember that one of the principles of Reiki is the attitude for gratitude. Any one you treat should be charged.

Charged in the sense, not of monetarily benefits. If the person taking Reiki from you cannot afford to pay you, and, you know he is incapable, request him to bake a cake for you, to cook any one dish for you. That person at a later date can run some chores for you, as, long as, the attitude of gratitude side is attained.

In the being when I first did my master/teachers degree, I charged US$40.00 per treatment. I even charged my students to teach Reiki.

I was told never to reveal the symbols. But, than I start thinking deeply.

- I reveal the symbols to people, who pay me, don't I.
- I revealed the secrets of attunements for people who did the Master/Teacher degree course with me, didn't I.

It this energy yours? OR Is this energy some private property?

Never. This is THE UNIVERSAL ENERGY.

Universal energy should belong to the UNIVERSE. To the people living in it. So, why not give this WONDERFUL GIFT to the people.

Most of the Reiki Master/Teachers I know charge the sky for teaching these techniques, TEACH but do not sell them. Teachers are not business people.

It is only education will always multiplies when given away. Just like a Smile, it will multiply and come back to you.

Hence, make sure, even if you have to take a pence or a cent for your treatment, accept it with the attitude of gratitude, but treat that person.

Hence, to complete your reach in the treatment of diseases, the Reiki 2 is a must.

REIKI 2

DAY 1
CHAPTER 3

ON THE ROAD TO SPIRITUALISM

I had traveled through umpteen modes of transport to reach the small place where the Master resided.

I was called in immediately.

The Master was seated in his meditation pose and an elderly man sat opposite him.

The conversation went like this:

"I wish to learn. Will you teach me?"

"I do not think that you know to learn" replied the Master.

"Can you teach me how to learn?" persisted the elderly guy

"Can you learn how to let me teach?" was the response from the Master.

Frustrated the man left. The Master looked at me and said:

"Teaching only takes place when learning does. Learning only takes place with you teach something to yourself."

REIKI 2

DAY 1
CHAPTER 4

THE THREE REIKI SYMBOLS

What Dr. Usui Mikao found in the Tibetan Sutras were 4 symbols. 3 of which are taught in the Reiki 2 class and the strongest one is taught in the Reiki 3A class. That is the reason the 3A Reiki is known as the Reiki Master Degree.

The Reiki Master cannot teach, because the 3A course does not teach you the techniques of attunements.

Of these 3 symbols - the first one is:

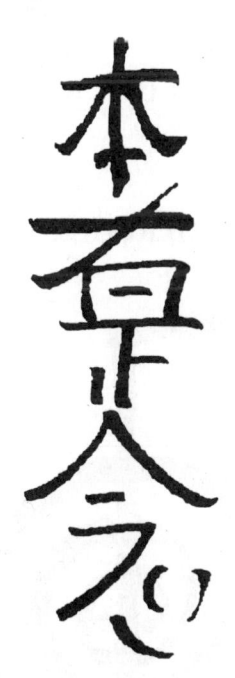

本
存
正
人
今
そ

HON SHA ZEH SHO NEN

This symbol is pronounced as "Hon (Hohhn) Sha (Shhaaah) Ze (Zay) Sho (Show) Nain (Nayn)

THE SECOND REIKI SYMBOL

The second Reiki Symbol is drawn as follows:

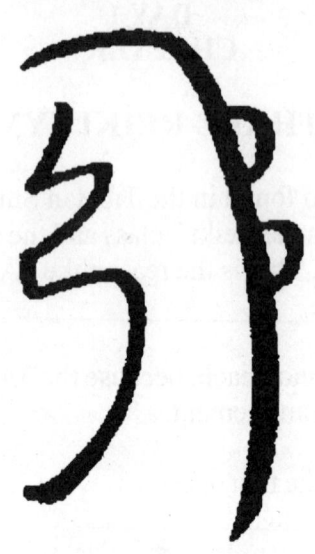

SEI HEY KI

This is pronounced as "Say Hay Ki"

THE THIRD REIKI SYMBOL

This symbol is drawn as follows:

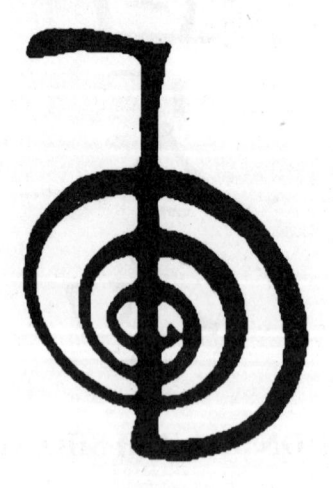

CHO KU RAY

The pronunciation is: "Cho (Chohh) Ku (Kooooo) Ray (as in "Ray")

REIKI 2

DAY 1
CHAPTER 5

WHAT TO DO WITH THESE SYMBOLS?

Doing the Reiki Seminars I conduct, I give the 3 symbols to my students; tell them to trace the first symbol with their forefinger. They do it. Over and over again. Then I tell them to trace this symbol from memory. Usually they do it on the first try, but I have never seen any student fail to draw this symbol in less then 10 minutes - maximum.

In the similar way the 2nd symbol and the 3rd symbol are taught. Compared to the 1st symbol, the 2nd & 3rd Symbols are very each to draw.

The 3rd symbol - "CHO KU RAY" and the 2nd symbol "SAY HAY KI" are mostly used for curing the cold areas.

Remember the 3 techniques to cure the cold areas? Yes, the shoveling and throwing bad energy into the cauldron, the treading and throwing into the universe and last but not the least, shoveling and throwing into a bucket with salt water.

These symbols are created for the same purpose. Now, when the cold areas are met with, you shovel and do the same as taught in Reiki 1, but at the same time, repeat the MANTRAS - either "CHO KU RAY" OR "SAY HAY KI".

Whichever Mantra enters your mind first should be repeated thrice.

MEANINGS & FUNCTIONS OF SYMBOLS
HON SHA ZE SHO NEN

HON	The centre, the essence, the source, the beginning, the start out of itself.
Sha	Shining
ZE	To walk in the right direction

SHO   The goal, aim, honest being
NEN   Silence, to be open in the deepest being of your nature (who you are)

The purpose of this symbol is to bring down the energy into your Heart Chakra, open the mind so that Reiki can operate beyond time and space.

Hon Sha Ze Sho Nen acts as a bridge for energy to flow. Though important particularly in Absent Healing, it is used always.

SEI HE KI

SEI   State of embryo, things which are invisible, source of external form.
HE KI   Root Chakra to be balanced.

Se He Ki breaks through or breaks down those, which are not in harmony. It breaks through our blockages and patterns on the aura level, emotional level and physical level and establish their harmony.

CHO KU REI

CHO   Curved sword (sickle), which draws a curved line.
KU   To enter something and produce wholeness, to produce space where nothing exists.
REI   Spiral, essence, mystical power, that which is not explanatory.
Cho Ku Rei Is the power symbol used for amplification of energy. It is a catalyst and activator.

Now, when you start giving Reiki to the patient, you start with the attitude of gratitude:

"I thank myself for being here,
I thank Reiki for being here,
I thank (name of the patient) for being here"

After this the first thing you do is place your cupped hands on the eyes of the patient. In Reiki 1 you just played the Reiki Cassette and awaited the sound of the bell. In Reiki 2, you start mentally drawing the first symbol through your 3rd eye chakra on the right eye of the patient. After the complete symbol has been drawn, repeat mentally, "Hon Sha Zay Sho Nayn" thrice.

Through your 3rd eye chakra, mentally draw the 2nd Symbol on the right eye. After the complete symbol has been drawn, repeat mentally, "Say hay Ki" thrice.

To the same with the 3rd symbol.

Now, repeat this exercise on the Left eye.

To summaries the above in a brief way:

The 3 symbols:

1. Hon Shah Zay Sho Nain
2. Say Hay Ki
3. Cho Ku Ray

Are to be drawn on every position you hand covers as shown in the table (see following page).

Points to remember:

- When I say a full set, it means each mantra drawn once, repeated thrice on a single position.
- On the table the number of positions are mentioned. A full set is to be done on each position.
- After the feet, do not forget to do the spirals.
- After the base of the spine is over, do not forget to do the chakra balancing, the caressing and the stroking.
- Draw each symbol from the third eye chakra to the hand in position and repeat the mantra mentally.

PARTS	POSITIONS
EYES	2
TEMPLES	2
EARS	2
FOREHEAD/BACK	2
BACK OF HEAD	1
THROAT CHAKRA	2
THYMUS / THYROID GLANDS	1
HEART CHAKRA	1
SOLAR PLEXUS	1
LIVER	1
LUNG TIPS	2
PANCREAS / SPLEEN	1
HARA	1
SPERMATIC CORDS (GENTS)	2
OVARIES (LADIES)	1
THIGHS (RIGHT)	1
THIGHS (LEFT)	1
KNEES (RIGHT/LEFT)	2
KNEES (RIGHT)	1
CALF (RIGHT)	1
ANKLE & SOLE OF FOOT (RIGHT/LEFT)	2
BACK - SHOULDERS	2
BACK - THYMUS & THYROID GLANDS	1
BACK - HEART CHAKRA	1
BACK - SOLAR PLEXUS	1
BACK – KIDNEYS	2
BACK – HARA	1
BACK - BASE OF SPINE	1

REIKI 2

DAY 1
CHAPTER 6

CHANTING OF THE SYMBOLS

After learning the Reiki symbols, I make it a practice to ensure that we do the following exercise:

- We sit in a circle.
- One student gets into the circle
- Excluding the one in the circle, all others start chanting "Hon Sha Zay Sho Nain"
- The student in the centre visualizes the symbol in the front of the 3rd eye chakra, while the others are chanting the first Mantra.
- The second Mantra is chanted "Say Hay Ki"
- The student in the centre visualizes the symbol in the front of the 3rd eye chakra, while the others are chanting the second Mantra.
- The third Mantra is chanted "Cho Ku Ray"
- The student in the centre visualizes the symbol in the front of the 3rd eye chakra, while the others are chanting the third Mantra.

We repeat this chanting with each student getting a chance to sit in the center and visualize.

At the end of the session, we ask about the experiences from the students.

REIKI 2

DAY 1
CHAPTER 7

INTRODUCTION TO MIND CONTROL HEALING

I have had a very good experience a few days ago. An Irish girl Wilma (name changed on request) paid me a visit. She had completed her course from another Reiki Teacher, and, odd things were happening to her. She was passing through a phase where she needed help and assistance.

She called her Reiki Teacher to help her during her healing crises. Unfortunately, she did not get any help from her Reiki Teacher.

I usually advertise in the local magazines, and, Wilma picked up my name from the magazine. She called me and asked for help. I asked her what help to you need?

She replied "I am in a trauma, tell me Mr. Mohan, ARE THE MIND AND THE BRAIN SAME THING?"

I replied in the affirmative, but she was not convinced. Then going over the books I found some articles on the brain, Meditation. Adding part of my knowledge to this I made an article for her which is presented to you:

Dear Wilma,

As requested by you. In return of your mind (Brain?) boggling question:

Are The Mind & The Brain same?

I am not an authority on this subject, neither is science my Forte. But, I have tried my best to answer your question as clearly and as honestly as possible.

Scientists have identified 4 basic types of brain (physical) waves:

1. *BETA*
2. *ALPHA*
3. *THETA*
4. *DELTA*

These correspond to the 4 levels of brain activity.

In Delta you produce brain waves of one half to four cycles per second (CPS) it is the zone of deep, unconscious sleep, a little known area of total unawareness.

In Theta, you produce from 5 to 7 CPS this is the zone of deep, comfortable sleep, an area of complete and utter satisfaction

In Alpha you produce from 8 to 13 CPS, alpha is the area of relaxing sleep and dreaming, sometimes also called the REM (rapid eye movement) because eyes flicker rapidly when you are dreaming.

In Beta, the outer conscious aware state, you brain produces waves of from 14 to 40 CPS. At the moment you are reading this article you are in beta.

The average person, at an average time, during an average day, is in the Beta area producing 21 CPS (actually the brain produces all 4 segments simultaneously; the amplitude, consistency, and frequency of waves determine the predominant area of activity).

Good health, intelligence, concentration, ease, pure genius lies in the area of brain wave production that falls below 19 CPS.

Psychosomatic problems are simply problems caused by the mind (psyche) getting in the way of the body (soma). By relieving the body of the problems of the mind through the alpha-generated separation of the psyche and soma, physical problems often resolve themselves.

An easy way to achieve the alpha state of ten cycles per second is through the meditative process. Meditation has a rhythm all its own, as does excitement, or anger, or for that matter any emotion that either stirs one up or calms one down. What meditation does is to slow down the brain waves and separate the mind from the body. This enables the mind to concentrate better, since it does not have to deal with the body's nervous system or emotional manifestations, or its reactions to outer and inner stimuli.

As far as the body is concerned, without the mind to harass it, the bodily intelligence can do its work. Its main job is to keep the cells in an energized balance so that it can be stabilized in a healthy condition. The major health benefit of meditation, then, is keeping the mind from interfering with the body so both may do their respective jobs - the body healing itself when ill and remaining healthy when healthy.

Your question has been answered above.

The "Mind" is defined as a "Psyche" (As per Webster - Psyche is defined as "Soul, Self, Mind") to go broader and deeper - into the meaning of "Soul & Mind", we have the following definitions:

Soul - The immaterial essence, animating principle, or actuating cause of an individual life. (Abstract - cannot be seen)

   The spiritual principal embodied in human beings. (Abstract cannot be seen)

   The quality that arouses emotions & sentiments. (Abstract - cannot be seen)

Mind - The element or complex of elements in an individual that feels, perceives, thinks, wills, and specially reasons (All Abstracts cannot be seen)

From the above it is conceived that the Mind is all respects in "Abstract" it does not have a body, while the brain is physical, it is present, and it can be seen.

Of course, the brain & the mind go hand in hand, encroaching on each other's territories so much, that it looks as if they are one and the same.

By sitting in mediation, the mind is controlled, this in turn controls the thoughts, then breathing is controlled and the nervous system relaxes, in lieu of which the brain also relaxes.

In conclusion of the above: It is my strongest belief that the Brain and Mind though they seem to be the same entity are not the same.

Hope I have been able to solve your dilemma.

Regards

DR. MOHAN MAKKAR Ph.D. (A.M.)

For any problems, you can always contact me on the usual phone nos., which you have.

Dated: 21/7/1997

I am sure you must have understood what is "Mind Control" from the above.

You can work wonders if you can visualize clearly with your 3rd Eye Chakra being the center of focus.

Once you have the art of controlling your thoughts, you can proceed with the alternate treatments:

Step 1:

- Pick up a patient you wish to treat.
- Analyze his/her sickness.
- Think how would a doctor heal this disease
- Think how you would treat this disease - memories it.

Step 2:

POINTS TO REMEMBER:

- Begin with visualisation.
- Go to your favorite place of relaxation.
- After relaxing a few moments, go to the Laboratory
- Wish each councilor individually.
- Discuss the problems with the councilors.
  As you already have the plan for treatment, see that all

equipments are ready.
- Bring the person wanting treatment into the mental frame of your 3rd eye chakra
- Ask permission to heal thus "By the power given to me by my Supreme Self, I request your permission to treat you of (give the name of the disease)"
- If the answer is "YES" call him to your Laboratory, where you go ahead with the treatment
- NEVER - NEVER - NEVER, treat a patient if permission by the Supreme Self is not granted or if you feel that the permission has not come through.
- On working near the chest or the heart area, create a mental clock, see it working, and then stop the clock. Proceed with treatment in the area. After the treatment is over. Re-start the mental clock.
- Always mentally wash your hands before and after the treatment.
- Do not talk with the patient.
- Depending on the chakra where the sickness is located, try and leave that particular colour in that area. If, you do not understand, do not ponder; just leave a shiny white light in the area.
- Be swift and accurate, do not hesitate. Withdraw if you wish to, or, if you feel nausea, but before withdrawing cover that area in white light before withdrawing.
- After the treatment cover the patient in white colour and encircle him/her in white light. Make the patient float in white light and leave him there, visioning that he is smiling and happy.
- Say thank you to the Supreme self of that person
- Say thank you to your higher self
- Say thanks you to your councilors - individually.
- Send the patient back to the place he had come from.

NOTE:

If you feel the person is having a chronic/major problem, do not let the person leave the laboratory. Leave the mental image under a post where he is immersed in the white light. Request your councilors to take care that the white light does not go off.

Also instruct your supreme self to carry out the treatment, which you have done, every 6 hours. What will happen is that though you may be consciously busy with your daily jobs, your subconscious mind will do the treatment every 6 hours.

Ensure you go to the laboratory and check on the patient at least every 24 hours.

If you are persistent and patient, RESULT WILL SURELY FOLLOW.

REIKI 2

DAY 1
CHAPTER 8

THE SOUND MEDITATION

During many seminars conducted by me, discussions have always followed with students who claim "I can NEVER sit in meditation with a taught entering my mind for more than 5 seconds"

Accepted.

During one such discussion, I asked the lady, "What if you sit in meditation for 5 full minutes and not a single thought enters your mind?"

The lady was perplexed. 5 MINUTES???

I smiled at her.

First of all I put on my Television and increased the sound to moderately high.
Next, I put on the FM Music
Then, my opened the windows of the drawing room. (As my house is located near the main road, we could hear the sound of moving vehicles very clearly)
Again, I took a piano from my daughter's toys and I started playing it.

There was a mixture of sounds in the room.

I told that lady and the other students in the room. " I give you all 5 minutes to count the number of sounds you hear" Then to bait them I added "Who ever can count the maximum number of sounds, will get a gift from me. The gift can be anything" then after a pause I added "Maybe a free Master degree Course"

Everybody was hooked.

I looked at my stopwatch. "START" I clicked my fingers.

There was silence in the room (by silence I mean - every one of my students stopped talking and closed their eyes in concentration - Meditation pose).

5 minutes slipped by. I was quiet. 6...............7.8 .... 9 ....10.

I stopped playing the piano.
I put off the FM Radio.
I put of the TV.
I closed the window.

Slowly, one by one, the students opened their eyes.

Everyone was smiling. A naughty mischievous smile on the face.

I looked at them and said "Okay - how many sounds"

"DAVID"
"48"

"MARC"
"17"

"ZUBAIR"
"72"

"MEENA"
"44"

"FLORA"
"84"

This was the lady who could not sit in Meditation for more then 5 seconds before a taught entered her mind.

"NIGEL"
"33"

"And," I continued, "May I asked if any one of you have any thoughts enter your mind"

Not a single one.

100% results.

I gave 50% fees off for the lady with the 84 sounds for that particular course.

Now, whenever I contact them asking them of their progress in Reiki & Meditation, I know that I have been successful with these students.

The sound meditation has become a most in thing.

REIKI 2

DAY 1
CHAPTER 9

A MEDIPIC HEALING EXERCISE

ARTHRITIS:

1. Contact subconscious mind of the sufferer and talk gently
2. Observe & identify all of the crystalline deposits on the bones of both hands
3. Mentally separate each joint and with a nail file or emery board, clean the bones of all crystal deposits
4. Before reassembling the joints, lubricate them well with golden oil; then saturate them with white healing energy as you fit them back in place.
5. See all fingers completely healed; all strong and supple once again, then slowly withdraw.
6. Do the same with knee joints, ankles and toes

(You can use pure sun's rays into the painful area and then paint it blue to soothe it)

REIKI 2

DAY 1
CHAPTER 10

SENDING LIGHT HEALING

- ℜ Select the person you want to be healed.
- ℜ Know the problem of the patient beforehand.
- ℜ Sit crossed legged in a meditation pose.
- ℜ Visualize the white circle over your Crown Chakra.
- ℜ Visualize the white light falling from the circle and covering your full body.
- ℜ Visualize yourself as transparent.
- ℜ Now, softly repeat the person's name you wish to be treated.
- ℜ Visualize the person in front of you.
- ℜ Visualize a light emanating from your 3rd Eye Chakra and falling at the problematic area of the person you are treating.
- ℜ Visualize the problem being solved.
- ℜ Visualize the light covering the person from head to toe.
- ℜ Visualize the fingers of his hands and toes taking out dark, oil type of liquid from his body.
- ℜ Hold this visualization till you see clear light passing through.
- ℜ Visualize him completely treated.
- ℜ Request the person to return back and inform him that he is now completely healed.
- ℜ Visualize you are coming back to your original self.
- ℜ Visualize the white circle diminishing and vanishing.
- ℜ Relax for a few moments before opening your eyes.

IT IS GUARANTEED THAT THROUGH THIS EXERCISE YOU CAN TREAT AND CURE MANY OF THE AILMENTS IN A

REIKI 2

DAY 1
CHAPTER 11

VISUAL MEDITATIONAL EXERCISE
THE UNIVERSAL BANK

- Φ Do the breathing technique and reach the Alpha Level
- Φ Goto your favorite place of relaxation (Your Sanctuary)
- Φ Relax for a few minutes - fly if you wish, go visiting your relatives/friends
- Φ Just relax
- Φ After you have relaxed, close your eyes and repeat the following words "By the power given to me by my higher self, I wish to go to THE UNIVERSAL BANK."
- Φ Feel yourself traveling.
- Φ Open your eyes (visualize) and you will find yourself in front of a building on which is written "THE UNIVERSAL BANK"
- Φ Climb the steps.
- Φ Start walking towards the doors.
- Φ Do everything at a leisurely pace.
- Φ Push the door inwards
- Φ You come across a single counter, which is being attended by a beautiful female (always visualize the opposite gender).
- Φ See her looking at you and smiling.
- Φ "Good Morning, Sir" she says
- Φ Reply in sweet tones "Good Morning to you"
- Φ "Can I help you?" she asks you.
- Φ Repeat the following words "Yes, I want to withdraw US$1,000,000.00 (or any figure you wish to withdraw)"
- Φ "One minute Sir" she says and opens up a drawer to give you a bland banker's cheque. "Can you fill this in?" she asks
- Φ Fill in the amount you wish to withdraw. Be confident. Be assured. This is the Universal Bank - you ask and it shall be yours. After filling in the cheque and signing it, hand it over the counter

to the lady.
- Φ Visualize her reading and requesting you to hold on.
- Φ Visualize her enter the cabin on the other side of the room.
- Φ Visualize her bringing in a leather suitcase with the cash.
- Φ Visualize her handing over the same to you.
- Φ Visualize you accepting the suitcase with the case and checking for authencity.
- Φ Visualize yourself thanking the lady and wishing her a good day and leaving the bank.

Come out of the Universal Bank and thank the bank for making your realization come true.

Repeat the following words - "By the power given to me by my higher self, I wish to return to my favorite place of relaxation."

Visualize yourself in your favorite place of relaxation.

Come back to your physical self whenever you want to do so.

REIKI 2

DAY 2
CHAPTER 1

ABSENTEE HEALING

On this side of the globe, we live far away from our Country, from our family, relatives & friends.

The only contact being e-mails, (which is rare) Postal Letters & Telephone calls. Of course we do miss our families and friends.

The only major burden on our shoulder is the 24 hours rattling of the chatterbox mind ... so, how's your family? So, how's your family? So, how's your family? This goes on and on and on and on, till people go berserk.

Can we control this rattling? Yes, if we know the mind control technique we can, but, also, if we think deeply on this question of "So, how's your family?" We can smile and say "In excellent health" the rattling will automatically stop.

But, how do we get that confidence, how do we justify the answer "In excellent health"

It simple, from our favorite place of relaxation, we can go to our home towns and as a casual visitation, without touching anything, without speaking we observe everyone and everything, then we quietly return to our favorite place.

During our above visit if we have seen any of our family members/relatives/friends who are not in perfect health, we can treat them from our house or from the favorite place itself.

Here, comes the importance of the Absentee Healing Technique, which is categorized in two:

1. The Short Form of Reiki
2. The Long Form of Reiki

Also, these techniques can be used for healing your friends and colleagues who cannot be reached immediately.

I wish you all good luck and again assure you that these are tried techniques where results have been achieved over and over again.

REIKI 2

DAY 2
CHAPTER 2

THE SHORT FORM OF REIKI

Okay, this is where we start Reiki in a different form. Can any one tell me why the short form of Reiki??

"...."

"Prakash?"

"Maybe, due to the constriction of time, this Reiki is taught," said Prakash dubiously.

"Right, you have hit the nail at the first shot. Let's take an example. You are a full-fledged Reiki Channel, unlike the ones who have just learnt to give Reiki on the 6 or 12 positions of the body.

"Just think, you are traveling on the bus, and, you see a cute little girl, who is crying away to glory, only to find that this baby has a severe tooth ache. What you cannot do is give her a full Reiki, which will take 1 hour 18 minutes. At this time, the short form of Reiki will help.

"Just try to become friendly with the child, repeat the Attitude ot Gratitude fast, than casually place your hands on the area of pain and start drawing the symbols - The Hon Sha Ze Sho Nen, The Say Hay Ki & The Cho Ku Ray, draw each symbol once and repeat it thrice. Give Reiki in the same position for 10 to 15 minutes.

"Believe me the child will be relieved, but, she had to get Medical attention fast."

"This was in person. But, what if the person is not there. Someone you know is suffering from some pain in the body, and, you know you do not have the time to give a full body treatment, what do you do?

"Yes, you give the Absentee healing - well, here is what you do"

1. Say the attitude of gratitude
2. Draw 1st, 2nd & 3rd symbols in your 3rd Eye Chakra
3. Cover yourself in white light.
4. Visualize the person you want treated, cover him/her in white light
5. Draw 1st, 2nd & 3rd symbols in the patient's 3rd Eye Chakra
6. Draw 1st, 2nd & 3rd symbols in the patient's Heart Chakra
7. Draw 1st, 2nd & 3rd symbols in the areas of pain (diseased parts) of the patient
8. Keep contact for 2 to 3 minutes
9. Close the process by drawing 1st, 2nd & 3rd symbols in your 3rd Eye Chakra

REIKI 2

DAY 2
CHAPTER 3

THE REIKI BOX

What's a Reiki Box??

I call it the MAGIC BOX.

This Reiki/Magic box has shown me many miracles with many of my students.

"Miracles?? Box??? I do not understand Sir??"

"Okay, I will try to make you understand"

The Story of Vishaal -

It was 0930 p.m. I was preparing to sleep when the telephone rang. I jerked and picked up the phone. It was from a Mr. Kodikal. "Mr. Mohan, I have your reference from Gulf News" he said "my wife is suffering from Chronic Arthritis and deformation has started, let us ask you - do you think she can be treated?"

I gulped - Chronic Arthritis? Deformation? I had never taken a case of this serious nature before. I closed my eyes and asked for permission from my Higher Self, I asked for guidance and out came another question "How long has she been suffering"

"8 years" a simple two words answer

"What's her age?" I queried

"63 years"

"Wow" I muttered under my breath.

"Well?" Mr. Kodikal was waiting for my answer

"Where do you live my Kodikal?" I asked

He replied by giving the location of his house.

"I am coming, now" I said. Kept the phone on the cradle and changed my clothes. Within 20 minutes I was at Mr. Kodikal's house - looking at a frail lady, in a wheel chair.

I gave her a Reiki session on the spot mixing this with visualization exercises, leaking out the pain from the knee joints, elbow and wrists. After about 45 minutes, I looked at her. She was smiling. The pain had reduced.

I looked at Mr. Kodikal.

"She will walk" I was confident.

"How long will it take?" he asked.

"I cannot give the period, but, your son has to come and learn Reiki from me. I will appoint 2 of my students who are Reiki Masters to give treatment twice daily. You pray we serve. Leave results to nature."

"Okay" Mr. Kodikal replied "My son will be coming in for the classes, when are they?"

"Tomorrow" I replied, the added "What's your son's name?"

"VISHAAL"

Anuradha - the lady's name is now completely cured. She walks around without any support of a human or walking stick. Her Chronic Arthritis has almost vanished, thanks to 2 of my most brilliant students - Mr. Narayan & his wife Mrs. Nagratna.

VISHAAL - has been working very hard at his job. When I taught the Reiki Box in the classroom, he refused to accept this foolish method, stating that Boxes cannot do miracles. But, then he put in an affirmation in the box, which read, "I am promoted as a Manager" and put in a date.

Now, it so happened, that during that time, a vacancy did arise for the post of a Manager, but, as he was too good at his present job, the General Manager, did not deem fit to take him out of his present job and upgrade him as a Manager.

That day Vishaal called me and challenged me that he could never get the job, whatever I did. I insisted that this vacancy had risen just because of the Affirmation in the Reiki Box and this vacancy was for him. "Don't give up, keep giving Reiki to the Box for one more month, believe me, Vishaal, this vacancy is for you - YOU WILL GET PROMOTED."

Vishaal shrugged away. But, promised to be a good boy and continue giving Reiki to the Reiki Box.

I almost forget about it, when (I think it was about 21 to 22 days after our meeting), I was cooking when the phone rang. I picked up the phone to hear Vishaal's exited voice

'MR. MOHAN - I GOT IT!!!!"

'WOW!!!" I shouted with glee. "You have done it, I told you, and this vacancy was for you."

Now, Vishaal is working as a Manager, whilst another affirmation is already in the Reiki Box for another promotion in the coming 18 months. WILL HE GET IT?? Well, it is for you to decide.

"Mr. Mohan, can you tell us what this Reiki Box is?" asked Geeta impatiently.

I smiled. It is always the case. AAAAAH - The Reiki Box.

Well, here it comes.

The Reiki Box is nothing but an ordinary soapbox. This can be activated with the following method:

1. Say the complete attitude of gratitude (For attitude and for gratitude, I thank myself for being here, I thank Reiki for being here, I thank the Reiki Box for being here)
2. Cover self with white light
3. Hold the Box in both your hands
4. Give symbols to yourself - (the 1st, 2nd & 3rd) from 3rd Eye
5. Give symbols to the Reiki Box - (the 1st, 2nd & 3rd) from 3rd Eye
6. See Reiki Box covered in white light for about 2 to 3 minutes
7. Close with 3 symbols - (the 1st, 2nd & 3rd) from 3rd Eye (this closes Reiki Box)
8. See Reiki Box covered in white light about 2 to 3 minutes
9. Close with 3 symbols - 1st, 2nd & 3rd) from 3rd Eye (this closes self)

YOUR REIKI BOX IS NOW ACTIVATED. NOW, YOU HAVE TO PUT IN AFFIRMATIONS IN THIS BOX.

"What are Affirmations?" I put in a general question to the class.

Of course, like most of the times, silence follows.

"AN AFFIRMATION IS AN INTENTION WHICH IS POSITIVE, PERFECT CONTINUOUS TENSSE I.E. YOU SEE ANY FUTURE EVENT HAPPENNG HERE AND NOW"

e.g. "Day by day in every way, I am feeling better and better and better"

We have the Reiki Box ready; we are now looking for the contents of the Reiki Box - which are the affirmations. Here are some of the rules for the REIKI BOX.

CONTENTS OF REIKI BOX:

1. The Reiki Box should include only 1 affirmation on one sheet of paper
2. Intentions should be positive, perfect continuous tense. i.e. you see any future event happening here and now.
3. All intentions should be as positive affirmations
4. For depression ask yourself the question "How do I feel?" Write the opposite (e.g. "How do I feel?" "I feel I am not being loved as I

should be" Affirmation will be "I am being loved and respected")
5. Cleaning of Reiki Box is essential as and when the intentions are fulfilled.
6. Uncleared intentions - if your intentions are not fulfilled on the given date, re-write them with dates
7. Write affirmations, which are nearer to your heart and not nearer to your ego.
8. You can put your own intentions, your friends/relatives intentions also.
9. You can put stamp/passport sized photos for healing in the Reiki Box
10. Invite friends intentions in Reiki Box or put in positive affirmations and let your friends sign themselves with date of fulfillment
11. YOU NEED NOT KNOW ALL THE INTENTIONS OF THE REIKI BOX.
12. The Rciki box can be of any material - the best is which appeals to your eyes.
13. Keep this Reiki Box in a clean and safe place (privacy is a must)
14. Give Reiki to the Reiki Box twice daily for approximately 2 to 3 minutes each time.

Most of my students claim that many of their dreams have been realized and they are very happy with this technique, which is unique.

TRY IT - IT MAY CHANGE YOUR LIFE FOR THE BETTER.

SOME OF THE AFFIRMATIONS

- I AM IN PERFECT HEALTH
- I AM FINANCIALLY STABLE
- I AM PROSPERING EVERY MINUTE
- I SEE EVERY NEGATIVE POINT WITH A POSITIVE VIEW
- I LOVE EVERYONE AROUND ME
- I AM BECOMING VERY PATIENT
- THOSE SURROUNDING ME ARE IN PERFECT HEALTH
- MY SENSE OF PERCEPTION IS INCREASING
- MY ATTITUDE TOWARDS EVERYONE IS BROTHERLY

- ♥ I LOVE LIFE IN EVERY FORM
- ♥ DAY BY DAY, IN EVERY WAY, I AM BECOMING BETTER & BETTER & BETTER
- ♥ DIVINE LOVE IS GUIDING ME AND I AM ALWAYS TAKEN CARE OF
- ♥ EVERY DAY I AM GROWING MORE FINANCIALLY PROSPEROUS
- ♥ EVERYTHING I NEED IS COMING TO ME EASILY & EFFORTLESSLY
- ♥ I ALWAYS COMMUNICATE CLEARLY AND EFFECTIVELY
- ♥ I AM LOVABLE AND A LOVING PERSON
- ♥ I AM ALWAYS IN THE RIGHT PLACE AT THE RIGHT TIME, SUCCESSIVELY ENGAGED IN THE RIGHT ACTIVITY
- ♥ I AM AN ACTIVE CHANNEL OF CREATIVE ENERGY
- ♥ I AM DYNAMICALLY SELF-EXPRESSIVE
- ♥ I AM LEARNING TO LOVE AND ACCEPT MYSELF AS I AM
- ♥ I AM NOW ENJOYING EVERYTHING I DO
- ♥ I AM RICH IN CONSCIOUSNESS AND MANIFESTATION
- ♥ I AM TALENTED, INTELLIGENT AND CREATIVE
- ♥ I AM VIBRANTLY HEALTHY AND RADIANTLY BEAUTIFUL
- ♥ I AM WHOLE IN MYSELF
- ♥ I AM TRUE TO MYSELF
- ♥ I LOVE MYSELF
- ♥ I AM RESPONSIBLE FOR MY OWN WELL BEING

You can, re-write the above affirmations in your own handwriting and place them in the Reiki Box. Moreover, daily reading of the

REIKI 2

DAY 1
CHAPTER 4

ON ROAD TO SPIRITUALISM
WHEN BUDDHISTS MEDITATE

(Guided Meditations, Explorations & Healings by Stephen Levine)

When human beings meditate. They sometimes close their eyes. And feel this body. A flickering field of sensations. A tingling, hot and cold, Gravity here and there.

And attend to the breath. At the belly or nostrils. Choose one and stay there five years.

Not the thought of the breath. But the sensations accompanying. Each inhalation. Each exhalation.

The beginning. The middle. The end. Of each in-breath. And the space between. Where thinking wriggles free.

The beginning. Middle. And end. Of each out-breath

And the space between. And thought. And the space between thoughts.

Returning to the breath. Just sensation breathing otse;f/Sensations sensing themselves. Floating in space.

Even some idea of who. Is doing all this. Floats by. Just another bubble

Another thought thinking itself. Mirroring like Escher. The fragile moment. Vanishing in space.

Returning to the breath "like a devotee. Who has broken a vow. A thousand times". And returns unruffled. Once again.

Watching thoughts. Think themselves. One into the next. Beginning momentarily to exist. And dissolving. Even such notions as impermamnence. Passing in the flow.

Observing feeling arise. Uninvited. Unexpectedly impersonal. Non one to blame. Or be blamed only. Just rope burns. From grasping to change.

And return to the breath again. Awareness making the old. Brand new.

Content dissolving into process.

Process floating in space.

Watching consciousness dream. Self and the world. Constantly creating more. Of there less to be.

We seek only to discover. That what is sought. Leaves the seeker far behind.

We are what we are looking for, For lack of a larger term, God.

REIKI 2
DAY 2
CHAPTER 5

THE LONG FORM OF REIKI

As stated earlier, most of the times it is a must that a full form of Reiki has to be given to a person who is not in your presence.

For this, you have to give the Long Form of Reiki, which can be divided into two groups.

Group 1 is very easy.

To start with please remember, the person you are sending Reiki to, be in bed or at least at home. Call the person up and confirm the person is at home. (Reiki seems to make people dizzy at times - unfortunately if the person is driving - complications may arise due to your giving Reiki at that time - as accidents can occur)

As we do the self-healing on ourselves, this type of long healing is done the same way. The only difference being the following words:

First you declare your body to be (the person's name you are treating):

"I declare my body to be Mr. Xxxxxxxx's body.

"I thank myself for being here"
"I thank Reiki for being here"
"I thank Mr. Xxxxxxxx's for being here"

Start, as you would do the self-cleansing technique.

After completing the full Reiki (26 positions) undeclare yourself as follows "I declare this body to be my own Mr. (your name) body"

Group 2:

Is to be done as follows:

- Say the attitude of gratitude
- Draw the 1st, 2nd & 3rd symbols on your 3rd Eye
- Cover yourself in white light
- Now imagine the patient whom you are about to give Reiki
- Cover the patient in white light
- Draw the 1st, 2nd & 3rd symbols on the patients 3rd Eye & Heart Chakras
- Declare the front portion of your Right Thigh is (name of the patient) front body
- Give Reiki to your Right Thigh as you would given Reiki to any person's front body (all 19 positions)
- Do the spirals - and lock the energy
- Now, declare the left portion of your thigh to be the patients back side of the body
- Cover the 7 points
- Close with Chakra Balancing
- Do the stroking
- Do the caressing

This completes the complete. Absentee Healing Method of Reiki.

REIKI 2

DAY 2
CHAPTER 6

THE MANY FACES OF REIKI

Reiki has other faces also:

Like you can healing the struggles in your life, release the tensions that you are going through, loosen the auras in your body (this is very helpful for depression cases), if you re not being healed, Reiki can again help you.

Do not worry if you do not find time to heal, whilst on bed, programme Reiki to be sent to anyone at any time on any given date, you can create future with Reiki, Heal the Dead if you feel you want to. If you are an introvert and are shy of people, why not try the Mental Method of Healing??

Shall we start??

♥ **HEALING OF STUGGLES:**

If you feel you can relax, relax.
Else do the breathing technique - Remember 4 in, 4 hold, 4 out and 4 hold.
You will feel relaxed.
Now, mentally scan your body and see where the pain is accumulating
Draw the 3 symbols on that area.
Place your Reiki hands on that area till you feel peaceful

♣ **HEALING OF TENSIONS**

Relax by the above method &/OR breathing technique
Look at the tension, which absorbs much of your time and energy.
Declare the same to your friend whom you trust, if not, write down this tension on a clean sheet of paper.
Give white light to this paper

Draw the 3 symbols on this paper
Visualize the tension being dissolved.

♣ AURA LOOSENING

Aura loosening is done when the patient is in a state of depression. The process is similar to pulling the blocks.

REIKI 2

DAY 2
CHAPTER 7

ENERGY CIRCULATION EXERCISE

During the 21 days of self-treatment, it is possible that you feel acute pain on your back in the Hara/Root Chakra region or enhanced sexual urge. This is indicative that the Kundalini has been touched and at this stage if you do not want to have sexual inter-course, you can transform this energy to higher consciousness by doing the Energy Circulation Exercise, as per the chart provided.

1. Lie on your back with your knees raised and feet touching the ground.
2. Feet should be slightly apart with hands at your sides, palms up.
3. Close your eyes.
4. Imagine a black ball (the size of a gold ball) on your genitals
5. With every in going breath tie the ball with the breath
6. With every out going breathe pull the ball upwards towards our Crown Chakra, turning the black ball into white.
7. The ball should be thrown out from the Crown Chakra only at the 36th breath and at this time the ball should be completely white.
8. Should the ball slip back, re-start the count.

Good Exercising.

REIKI 2

DAY 2
CHAPTER 8

ABSENTEE HEALING - PRACTICAL EXERCISE

Pneumonia/wet-cough/asthma (wheezing)

1. Centralize yourself

2. Go to alpha

3. Go to your laboratory

4. Discuss the case with your councilors

5. Call the patient

6. Open the chest area

7. See the Phlegm/dust on the lungs.

8. For the Phlegm start the draining with 2 taps on the bottom of each lung. See Phlegm been drained away. For the dust vacuum out the same.

9. Once the lungs are emptied out, you can start the healing process by visualizing healing body tape covering sore areas and soothing, pain-removing oil being passed through and around all the tubes, (also effective for bronchitis) as well as over the inner lining of the lungs themselves.

10. Ensure that throat, bronchial tubes and lungs all healed and functioning normally as you give them a final shot of white energy and instruct the inner mind to repeat the procedure at an interval of 12 hours until a relapse is no longer likely.

REIKI 2

DAY 2
CHAPTER 9

VISUAL MEDITATION EXERCISE
LET'S TRAVEL

During the classes held on regular basis, students just snigger behind my back whispering that it is a hotchpotch idea, a play of mind, that any one can be sitting in a comfortable position and his ethereal body can travel hundreds of miles in a matter of a few seconds.

See friends and relatives and then return with information on what it has seen and heard - HOW CAN THIS BE TRUE? - They ask.

Well, it is simple.

The Physical body, which functions - is made up of 5 materials, Earth, Water, Ether, Air & Fire. Even the Bible says "Dust thou art and to dust thou shall return"

But what about the ethereal body??? What about the Soul???

"Thou shall rise after death," says the Bible - "This 'THOU' is the ethereal body, which comes from the word ETHER and is known also as the twin soul. This Twin Soul or the ethereal body is attached to the physical body with a golden chord. At the time of death this cord is detached from the body and then the ethereal body in which the Chakras and the Soul also exist, cannot attach itself to the body again.

At this stage, the ethereal body remains in the zone as per their Karmas and the Soul - also known, as the BLUE PEARL is re-born. One of the few theories explains that this soul is immediately put in the womb of a woman who is in the 3rd month of pregnancy, and, for the next 6 months this soul - in the mother's womb is shown the life he/she has led.

The pure nectar of this explanation is the ethereal body and the Golden Cord attached to it with the Physical body. The Cord is extendable and though attached to the physical body, can travel millions of miles - in either direction. This type of travels is also known as ASTRAL TRAVELS.

During the Astral Travels you can perform miracles, which will be known only to you. You can visit friends and relatives.

Our purpose of visiting is to detach the ethereal body from the physical body and request it to visit any place we choose.

Here is what we do:

First we go to our favorite place of relaxation.

1. Relax for some time.
2. Repeat the following words "By the power given to my higher self, I request my Ethereal body to some in front of me"
3. (Here you may see a grayish/bluish substance in front of you - at this stage you will be unable to move any of your body parts, clinically you may be dead at this time, the pulse rate may have dropped to 3 to 5 beats/second)
4. When you see your Ethereal Body in front of you, request this body to visit any of your relatives, friends any one you wish
5. Within seconds you will feel you are there - in the house you wished to be.
6. (Two things are very important here - (a) Try to see the calendar and time in that house - make a mental note of date and time)
7. Take a note of all surroundings. You will be unable to touch anything. Everything you see may be opposite of what you may have seen in the physical body. For example, when you are facing the kitchen the bathroom door may be on the right hand side (physical), but, in the Astral level the bathroom door will appear on the left hand side. See the bed sheets, the table covers, the mats, cutlery, people, their clothes, colors on the walls every possible detail you can gather.
8. Request your ethereal body to come back to your physical body. It should be back within seconds.
9. Be careful, not to get up immediately.
10. Lie down still, relaxed.
11. After a few minutes, slowly open your eyes assess how you are

feeling. If you are feeling fresh get up, if not, close your eyes again and relax for a few more minutes, it may be due to the ethereal body not coming back to the physical body completely.
13. When you are up and about, try to recollect what had happened and what you had seen. Jot everything down. Do not rely on your memory. These thoughts sooner or later disappear.
14. Write a letter to the person whose house you have visited giving descriptions, be vague and brief, just say you had a dream and you saw....
14. DO NOT BE SURPRISED IF YOUR FRIEND ANSWERS WHAT YOU SAW WAS 100% CORRECT.

REIKI 2

DAY 2
CHAPTER 10

ACTIVATING YOUR ETHEREAL BODY

- Sit/Lie down in a comfortable position.
- Take a deep breath to the count of 4 filling in your breath to the navel. Stop your breath to the count of 4. Breathe out to the count of 4 from your mouth.
- Repeat till you feel completely relaxed.
- Visualize a white circle over your Crown Chakra.
- Bring this white circle towards your Root Chakra from the spinal column.
- See the White circle being attached to your Root Chakra.
- See the root chakra rotating and emanating Red Light.
- Move the white circle to the sexual chakra and attach the same to it.
- See the sexual chakra rotating and see an orange light flow out of the chakra.
- Move the white circle to the solar plexus chakra and attach the same to it.
- See the solar plexus chakra rotating and throwing out pale yellow light.
- Now, move this white circle to your heart chakra and attach it.
- See the heart chakra rotating and green light splash in circles.
- Move the white circle to your throat chakra and attach it.
- See the throat chakra rotating. See a light blue light coming out of the throat chakra.
- Move the white circle to your 3rd Eye Chakra and attach the same to it.
- See the 3rd Eye Chakra rotating and emanating an indigo light.
- Bring the white circle of light to the Crown Chakra. Attach this white circle to the Crown Chakra and see the Crown Chakra activated. See a Violet light emerge from the crown chakra.
- Bring the white circle to your front side and attach it to the 3rd Eye Chakra. See the 3rd eye chakra rotating and give out an indigo colored light.
- Slip this white circle into your mouth and from over the soft spot

above the tongue into the throat chakra. Attach this circle to your throat chakra. See the throat chakra rotating and giving out a light blue light.
- Bring down the white circle to your heart chakra. Attach the white circle to the heart chakra. Visualize the heart chakra giving out green light.
- Bring the white circle down to the solar plexus chakra. Repeat above and visualize the solar plexus chakra give out a light yellow light.
- Bring the white circle down to your sexual chakra. Repeat above. Visualize an orange colour light come out from the sexual chakra.
- Bring the white circle to the center of your root chakra. See the white light evaporate.
- Now, see all the chakras rotating from the root chakra to the crown chakra from your spinal column and from the crown chakra to your root chakra from the front side of your body. You will only see a white colour light emanating at a very high speed.
- Increase the speed. As you increase the speed you will see another body, which is attached to your physical body, start to move. Move this body, which is also of white/grayish to your left and right side.
- Move this ethereal body in front of you. You can see yourself now. Let this ethereal body float to the roof. See yourself lying down.
- Slowly, let the ethereal body come back to your body and settle down properly.
- Visualize the white circle slow up its speed and finally stop.
- Put both your palms on your eyes.
- Open your eyes under your palms.
- Relax and open your eyes.

REIKI 2
DAY 2
CHAPTER 11

THE YIN & THE YANG PAIN KILLERS

This is a unique technique yet a simple one.

How did I come across it?

Well, one day, it so happens that I was reading a book, in this book, I came across the following story of a sage, a Sufi, a saint.

It so happened that this saint was traveling by a train with his disciples, when the train stopped at a particular station. An old man saw this saint and invited him for dinner.

This old man was so poor that many a times, he found it difficult even to feed himself. But, somehow, the saint accepted the invited much to the annoyance of his disciples.

After having the meal at the old man's home, the saint saw that the young girl, who served him, was full of white marks on the body.

Now, the saint wanted to return back and continue the journey, but not before repaying the old man for all the love he got from him.

So, he took the girl's hands in his hands, and lo & behold!!!! The saint was full of white marks, but the girl had become completely clean. She had turned into a very beautiful maiden.

The disciples were perplexed. But, quietly the saint went out of the house, and, sat under a birch tree, and, again the disciples saw a miracle, the birch tree took the white marks on it and the saint was cleared of the white marks (Rune Power?????) And after a few minutes the tree itself was free from the white marks.

After reading this story, I pondered for weeks over this. Whilst sleeping at night, I requested my higher self to take me to the place and time as a silent witness to see that had happened in that village.

In the morning when I woke up, I had pieces of images in my thoughts. That day, a very fat lady walked in to my house for treatment. She had problems with her left elbow joint, which pained very severally.

A taught rose in my mind, why not try this method of the saint?

I took her hands in my hand and told her what to do, giving her the "click" point, which would indicate the pain had vanished.

I was thrilled when just after 3 minutes the "click" came.

I looked at her and smiled. "YES" she was puzzled. The pain had gone. What happened??

Here's the conversation after the click:

"What happened?"

"My pain's gone"

"Completely?"

"Yes" - there was still disbelief in her voice.

"Since when did you have this pain?"

"Last 3 years "pause, then" I have consulted many doctors, ayurvedics & homeopaths, but there has been no relief

"Who referred you to me?"

"Your student Bhavna" she replied.

I assured her that the pain would not return, and, if it does, please return back.

SHE HAS NEVER COME BACK.

But, 3 hours later, after the above treatment, I felt a severe pain in my left elbow. I ignored this pain, not knowing what it was.

Then +2 hours later, the pain became unbearable. I found tears rolling out of my eyes. What happened? I started recollecting my thoughts and found out that I had taken the pain away from that lady's elbow.

Suddenly, IT HIT ME!!!! Yes, I had taken the pain away from the lady, but what had I done with it. PUT IT IN MY BODY. So, the pain was till in my body. But, I had never let it out.

Immediately I sat in a meditation pose and after 15 minutes of meditation, I found complete relief in my left elbow.

From that day onwards, I have treated dozens of cases, where immediate relief is required with this technique, which I have name "The Yin & the Yang"

One more case I treated with this technique was a Mr. Mahesh. During the week end my family and a few friends were traveling in a car to attend a party. One of the occupants in the car was Mr. Mahesh. I could see his eyes were reddish and a friend of his (Mr. Prakash) was puffing into a handkerchief and putting that on his eyes.

On reaching the house, (a studio apartment), I saw Mahesh's eyes were completely red. I instantly knew it was Conjunctivitis. I took Mahesh in to the kitchen and kept my hands on his eyes. After a few minutes when I removed the hands, his eyes had cleared. The time was 12.15 a.m.

I did not have the place to throw away that diseased energy, so I with held it in me, for had I taken it away from me, it would be possible it could have gone to some one in that single room apartment. By 3.00 a.m. my eyes had gone completely red.

The guests in the house were shocked. They knew Mahesh had conjunctivitis, but, suddenly he was cleared of it and I had the same problem in me now. Mahesh explained that I had done something. They could not comprehend what had happened.

By 4.00 a.m. when we left the house, my eyes were watering profusely. My wife had to drive us back home. Once at home, I sat in the Meditation pose and within 30 minutes of meditation, my eyes had cleared and I was perfect again.

At 10.00 a.m. most of the guests came to visit me for they knew that I must be in tremendous pain. Again they were in for a shock. I was up and about and smiling.

They request I should teach them this technique, which of course I refused.

My question to them was this:

"Do you have enough love in you to take other people's pain in your body and suffer yourself? Remember, every time the pain cannot be washed away, some of it will always remain with you. Are you willing to suffer for others???? Yes, Christ did, but will you?

If yes, go ahead and go to the next chapter.

REIKI 2

DAY 2
CHAPTER 12

THE YIN & THE YANG - METHOD OF HEALING

The concept:

This treatment is based on the fact that pain is always black in color. This pain, can be either hard like a rock (Chronic pain), soft like a jelly - acute pain), or similar to cotton.

What we have to do is, hit this pain with a white light, which goes from our Right hand to the patient's left hand. This light travels at a very high speed hitting the black pain and smashing it, crushing it or melting it, which than travels through the patient's right hand and is then thrown in to your left hand. Which you retain it in yourself.

You have to indicate to the patient that:

1. He visualizes a white light falling from your right hand into his left hand.
2. Imagine this light traveling towards his shoulders and towards his right hand.
3. Hitting the pain and melting/breaking the pain into small sand like pieces
4. The pain, which is black in color passing with the force of white light into your left hand.
5. Till the patient does not feeling the white light fluently passing from his left hand to his right hand he will continue visualizing the white light hitting the black pain and the black pain giving way.
6. When the white light passes from his left to right hand, he has to press his left hand thumb on your left hand, indicating the session is over.
7. Wait for a few seconds and release the hands, which are clasped.

The pain is now in your hand, and, the patient is relieved.

What you have to do is this:

1. Sit in a meditation pose.
2. Visualize a white/golden/Electrical Violet light circle on your Crown Chakra.
3. See this light circle spinning - fast, faster, faster, faster - as it is spinning it is emitting the color, which is being poured over your Crown Chakra and into your third eye chakra.
4. As you visualize see this light passing from your 3rd Eye Chakra to your Throat, Heart, Solar Plexus, Hara, and Sexual & Root Chakras.
5. Visualize this light energy pass through your shoulder blades into your arms, elbows and thrust that black pain into your palms.
6. Visualize the black pain seeping out of your hands till a clear light does not pass through.
7. The balance energy will cover, protect and energize you keeping you completely fit.

Thank the energy for the miraculous healing.

REIKI 2

DAY 2
CHAPTER 13

SUMMARY

Congratulations!! You have now completed the Reiki 2 course.

Let's summary what we have learnt in Reiki 2 - first, we shall segregate the Mind Control and Reiki sessions:

In Reiki we have learnt:

1. The Symbols and their meanings. Also, we have learnt how many sets of symbols are to be drawn on each position.
2. We have learnt the Absentee healing method - where it is a must to ensure that the person you are healing is at home when the healing is being sent.
3. We have also learnt the Short Form of Reiki - which works miracles in a short duration - for this too; it is requested to ensure that the person you are healing is at home when the healing is being sent.
4. The Magic Box - officially named "The Reiki Box" you have to be very careful to ensure that the affirmations written by you are as taught to you in this chapter.
5. The Long form of Reiki - is a technique where you declare your 'Body' or 'Your thighs' (left & Right) to be the person you are healing, and, you have to give full Reiki inclusive of the spiraling, Chakra balancing, stroking & caressing. After which you have to undeclare your body or your thighs to be your own.
6. In the many faces of Reiki we have learnt different uses of Reiki.

In Visual Meditation we have learnt -

1. Sending Healing Light
2. The Universal Bank - the more you practice on this, the clearer your visualization the better chances will occur for realizing your dreams
3. In Let's Travel, continuous practice of this exercise sets about

your ethereal body to travel in different zones. But, do ensure that the telephone/s are kept off the hook; the mobiles & Pages are switched off and doubly ensure that you are not disturbed when you do this exercise.
4. In Activating your Ethereal Body we learnt how to loosen the auric body and how to travel. We have to take all the precautions of No. 3 - Let's Travel exercise.

We have also learnt The Sound Meditation and the Yin & the Yang pain Killers. Please do not practice the Yin & the Yang if you are sick or suffering from body aches in your body. Also do ensure that immediately as the pain is taken out of the patient's body, you sit in Meditation yourself and do the exercise taught in this chapter till you get full relief from the pain in your body.

REIKI

3A - THE MASTER'S DEGREE
CHAPTER 1

A DISCUSSION

Welcome to the Master's degree class.

We have achieved some direction in our life. Our life was a log floating in a stream with no direction. Wherever our life takes us we go. Our life was like a wild horse. No controls - like a car without a steering wheel.

Now, we have the steering wheel - REIKI.

We have taken the control of our wheel - the reins are in our hands and the wild horse has been broken. We are sitting on the log, which was floating aimlessly down the stream - all in all we have DIRECTION.

We are one of the few people in the world.

By doing this course, we shall become stronger.

Before that we have to assess what we have learnt.

- We have learnt Reiki - through which we can cure people with the Universal Energy by our hands.
- In Reiki we have learnt the short form & the long form of Reiki.
- We have taught the Reiki Box where we put in our affirmations.
- We have repaired our childhood.
- Most important - We have learnt to travel in any part of the world, visit anybody at any given time.
- We have our own favorite place of relaxation.
- We have our own laboratory for treatment and our own Councilors.
- We have learnt in part the technique of Metaphysical healing.
- We have learnt in part the technique of Mind Control healing.
- We have learnt to Meditate.
- AGAIN, MOST IMPORTANT - We have learnt to use the white

light to heal people, circumstances, and relations.
- We have learnt the 3 symbols, which made our world of Reiki more powerful.

Now, today we shall increase this power - we shall become Masters - THE REIKI MASTERS.

This is what we do. We say, we do not want this, and, do a hundred things too. Avoid not wanting that. But, if we turn our thinking and attitude and say "I want this" and create a desire to get that, and, do a hundred things to get that, we WILL GET WHAT WE WANT.

One of the 2 monks, just whisked her on his shoulders, stepped into the water and left her on the other side of the stream. The other monk was quiet. But the monks traveled a few miles, when suddenly the other Monk spat out "But why did you carry her?"

The first Monk smiled at his mate and said, "I carried her, I left her - that was it. But, you are still carrying her"

This is what our life is. We are carrying too many corpses on our shoulders. We have to many things in our life which we DO NOT WANT, and, the better part of our life is waster in dwelling in the "NO ZONE"

I recollected one more episode of a guy who went Para sailing. It was the first time he had jumped from the mountain and he was doing beautifully well, when suddenly the instructor below shouted - "Hey, you see that red car, don't go and bash in there"

That guy's attention was divided. He began searching for the red car below him. He saw the car and of course, he bashed into the car!!

REIKI

3A - THE MASTER'S DEGREE
CHAPTER 2

WHAT IS REIKI 3A?

Like the other Reiki sessions, this session is important. I wouldn't say important, but it is unique. Because, it will change you, change you to a better person, more understanding, and more loving, more caring.

Reiki 3 - discussions with the Master/Teacher brings you to a higher level of understanding the people around you. If someone comes to you, do not shoo that person away. DO NOT JUMP TO CONCLUSIONS.

Sometimes what the ears hear may not be the truth. Also, sometimes what the eyes see is ALSO NOT THE TRUTH.

Do not carry corpses on your shoulders. Let bygones be bygones. I remember a small story I had read about the 2 Tibetan Monks. These monks live a solitary life. They are not allowed to talk, beg, come in contact with the opposite sex etc. etc. etc.

Now, one day as these 2 monks were traveling they came upon a stream, which had to be crossed. The flow of the water was very strong. They saw a young girl, trying to step into the water, but, every time she tried to put her foot in, she stepped back, for the fear of being washed away in the stream.

This is drawn from the 3rd Eye Chakra on the area of the patient's body where the problem exists.

This is a very-very powerful symbol and brings results very quickly. Do not go on flaunting this symbol. Be serious in this area of treating people, as, you will be seeing too many people being healed and also a ratio of people being passed on to the land of no return.

I can just wish you GOOD LUCK.

REIKI

3A - THE MASTER'S DEGREE
CHAPTER 3

THE MASTER SYMBOL

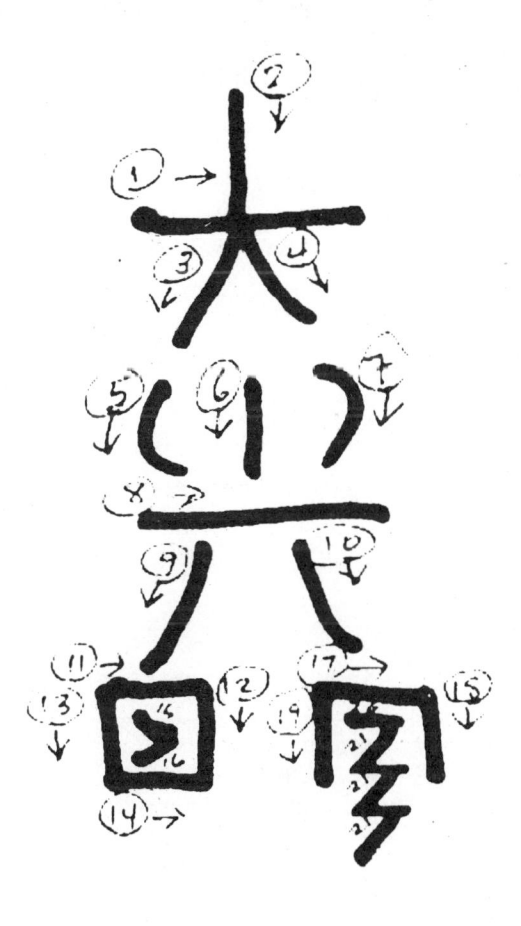

There are 3 parts in this symbol : The 1st one is "DAI" - Meaning "Great" :

The symbol is drawn thus :

The master symbol

On the whole "Dai Ku Mayo" - pronounced as "Dai Ku Mayo"

Meaning - "The Great White Light" - is drawn as follows:

This is drawn from the 3rd Eye Chakra on the area of the patient's body where the problem exists.

This is a very-very powerful symbol and brings results very quickly. Do not go on flaunting this symbol. Be serious in this area of treating people, as, you will be seeing too many people being healed and also a ratio of people being passed on to the land of no return.

I can just wish you GOOD LUCK

REIKI

3A - THE MASTER'S DEGREE
CHAPTER 4

DO YOU NEED REGRESSION?

What is regression?

Regression means "Progressive decline"

It is not necessary for everyone to undergo a regression or re-birthing course.

You have to take into consideration most of the following:

1. Your relationship with your family members
2. Your relationship with your friends/colleagues
3. Your relationship with YOURSELF
4. Your relationship with your work
5. Your relationship with each and every aspect of your life.

What we have to ask ourselves is:

Why is our relationship bad with one member of the family and good with the other member? Though, you may consider, you are very soft spoken and of a very milk nature where others are concerned.

They why the difference?

Have you ever thought, sometimes, you see a person whom you have never met before, and, instantly you have a bad taste in your mouth? Have you ever asked the question to yourself - Why do I feel this bad taste in my mouth? Why do I feel this hatred in me, I have never seen this person in my life before?

On the other hand, you a person for the first time, and bingo. You are in love with that person. Again, WHY?

Mainly, on the subject of regression, we take our present status. How is my relationship with my family members? Bad?? How is their relationship with me, good? If it is good, than something must be wrong with me. It is my fault.

Regression/Re-birthing are techniques which slowly and gradually take you into the past making you meet people and enabling you to see events wherein you have suffered and which has effected your present life.

Slowly, the teacher takes you backwards to your childhood and still more to your previous birth. Here you see your life, see the faces of the people and come back to the present life and recognize those faces. Then you make connections. All the way to the past and present, past and again to the present again and again and again. Till you know the relationship, the reasons.

The teacher explains and asks you to pardon those people who have harmed you. For, if you do not, you get them back into your next birth. By pardoning them, you complete your relationship with these people, paving a way for them to get out of your life never to return again.

So, if you think, that you love someone, and, still it is not working out, go for the regression/re-birthing and may be YOU WILL HAVE YOUR ANSWER - YOU
Never know.

REIKI

3A - THE MASTER'S DEGREE
CHAPTER 5

DO YOU LIVE BY THE ATTITUDE OF GRATITUDE WAY OF LIFE?

Let me ask you one question? No. Do not get fidgety; it's nothing that will embarrass you.

How many times in a day do you use the "F" word? Or say "Shit!"

I believe, it is most common to do so, say "Umpteen" times a day??

What is important to note is that when you say "S-h-I-t" all the emphasis are laid on the sound "SH" which takes out all the pressure from your head.

Similarly the "F" (pronounced = Fuh)

This air, which is let out in a short out bound breath, relieves you immediately and makes you feel comfortable. Most of the times, y you may notice that after using these types of vulgar, dirty words, which are the most in-things, especially amongst the teenagers, you feel relaxed.

So, it is not "SHIT" which is important. The word can also be "SHIP" because the emphasis is still the same "SH". Try it sometimes. You will achieve the same results and people around you may not catch on the word for a few days.

Similarly the "F" word should be changed to something like "Fut." instead of "F…" (Fut. means 'future')

Such other obscene words can be changed to words, which have goods meanings.

The exercise is simple; the implementation is hard - but not impossible.

This will take you to a stage of attitude of gratitude.

Whilst on the subject of attitude of gratitude, let me ask you another question. No, do not groan, every question I ask you will take you a step closer to making you a better person, a healthier person, physically, mentally & spiritually.

How many minutes a day to you give yourself?

Most of the answers I get from my students are : Not even a single.

How may minutes have nature given you in a day? Did you consider that?

24 hours/day x 60 minutes/hour = 1,440 minutes/day.

Out of these 1440 minutes/day how may·times do we say that you to the facilities available to us.

For instance saying thank you:

Saying thank you to each and every part of our body for working 24 hours of the day non-stop in order to keep us healthy and active.

- The sink in the kitchen for making our task easier by allowing us to wash the utensils on the spot.
- The gas cooker
- The TV Set
- The Sofa Set
- The dining table
- The Computer
- Our family members for making us feeling important
- Our boss for giving us a job, which feeds our family

The list is endless; it can go on and on and on.

This acceptance of gratitude will make you humble. Do not ever doubt that the nature, the body, the people, the things are not listening. They listen. They act. Everything, anything is ENERGY you too are ENERGY. For energy to energy. Thank it. Say "Thank you for. " and mean it.

Life will become easier. You will become a different person. You will notice in slow motion the changes, which will come over you.

The Armour of irritation will melt away, the ego will vaporize.

Peace will be your forte. Perfect health will smile at you as long as you are in this world.

Accept the problems, solve them, but, always "The Attitude of Gratitude" should be there to make our life one long happy journey.

REIKI

3A - THE MASTER'S DEGREE
CHAPTER 6

QUESTIONS & ANSWERS

I sincerely hope that you have completed the 3A course before answering these questions and do not refer to the notes again.

Once more, before answering these questions, ask yourself, "Have I done the 21 days cleansing?" If the answer is "YES" go ahead and attempt the questions. If the answer is "NO" do the self-cleansing first, then attempt the questions.

Remember, though I may not see you, I am with you and your answer will give me an insight into your experiences with REIKI. These are enough for me to know, if you are being honest with me.

Now, the questions:

1. After you finished the Reiki 3A Course, you did the 21 days self cleansing with the master symbol. What were your experiences?
2. How do you feel after completing this course?
3. What do you think of yourself as a whole person? State if you feel you have any more draw backs in your life?
4. Write about your drawbacks. I may be able to help you become one with yourself.
5. Remember, while giving Reiki to others at the 3A level, which is also known as the Master Level, you Motto should be "Let me lead you gently back to yourself" Why do you think this motto has been chosen.
6. When it is said "Let me lead you gently back to yourself" what comes to your mind?
7. How many people have you treated till date? Please write in full the names, their illnesses, and period of cure and if the results were positive.
8. What are your thoughts when you are treating people?
9. Do you charge fees from the people you are treating?
10. Do you live in the "Attitude of Gratitude" way?

ON THE ROAD TO SPIRITUALISM

- The Master once said "in the land of the spirit, you cannot walk by the light of someone else's lamp. You want to borrow mine, I'd rather teach you how to make your own."

- Then at another time Sometimes there would be a rush of noisy visitors and the Silence of the monastery would be shattered.

  This would upset the disciples; not the Master, who seemed just as content with the noise as with the Silence.

  To his protesting disciples he said one day, "Silence is not the absence of sound, but the absence of self."

- "How would spirituality help a man of the world like me?" asked the businessman.
  "It will help you to have more," replied the Master.

  "How?"

  "By teaching you to desire less"

- The disconsolate stockbroker lost a fortune and came to the monastery in search of inner peace. But he was too distraught to meditate.

- After he had gone, the Master had a single sentence by way of wry comment: "Those who sleep on the floor never fall from their beds."

- "I have no idea of what tomorrow will bring, so I wish to prepare for it."

  "You fear tomorrow not realizing that yesterday is just as dangerous."

REIKI

3B - THE MASTER / TEACHER
CHAPTER 1

PREPARING FOR AN ATTUNEMENT

In order to improve the results you receive during the attunement, a process of purification is recommended. This will allow the attunement energies to work more efficiently and create greater benefits for you. The following steps are a must if you need to prove yourself as the best student and achieve maximum results. Follow them if you feel to do so:

1. Avoid each non-vegetarian food for three days prior to attending the classes. These foods often contain drugs in the form of penicillin and female hormones and toxins in the form of pesticides and heavy metals that make your system sluggish and throw it out of balance.
2. Consider a water or juice fast for one to three days specially if you already are a vegetarian or have experience with fasting.
3. Minimize your use of coffee and caffeine drinks else stop completely. These create imbalances in the nervous and endocrine systems. Use no caffeine drinks on the day of the attunement.
4. Use no alcohol for at least three days prior to the attunement.
5. Minimize or stop using sweets. Do not each any chocolate.
6. Cut down on smoking or do not smoke the day you are attending the classes.
7. Meditate an hour a day for at least a week using the easiest meditation technique else speaks at little as possible.
8. Reduce or eliminate time watching TV, listening to Radio and reading newspapers.
9. Using time saved for quiet walks, spending time with nature and getting moderate exercises.
10. Give more attention to subtle impressions and sensations within and around; contemplate their meaning.
11. Release all anger, fear, jealousy, hate, worry, etc. Create a sacred space within and around you.
12. Use you Reiki guide (Your Reiki teach will guide you)

REIKI

3B - THE MASTER / TEACHER
CHAPTER 2

THE TECHNIQUE - ATTUNEMENT REIKI

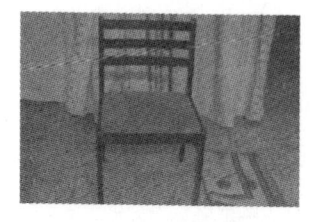

The instruments:
1. Chair
2. 2 Mat
3. Cymbals

I) Bring Reiki student into the room.

II) Make Reiki student sit as in the picture, with feet about 10" apart

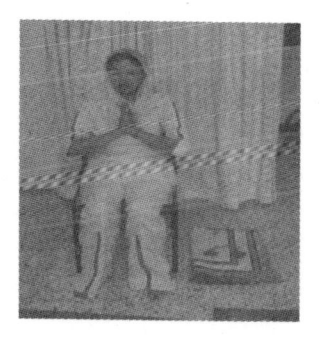

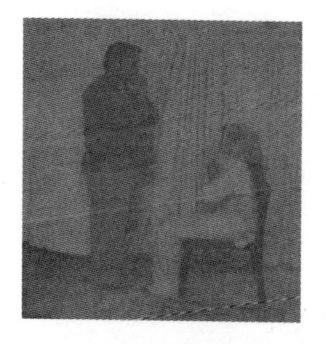

Stand in front of the student and joint both hands.

1. Go on your haunches (toes inwards)
2. Repeat mentally the following:
a. I thank myself for being here. I request my personality to step aside.
b. Continue repeating mentally "I think Dr. Usui for being here. I thank Dr. Hayashi for being here. I thank Mrs. Takata for being. I thank Mr. Makkar for being here. I thank (insert all your family members' names here).
c. I thank my Soul Leaders for being here.
d. I request my physical self to step aside (visualize your physical stepping aside)
3. I surrender and let go.

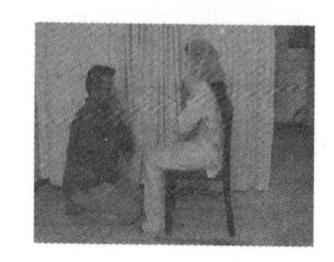

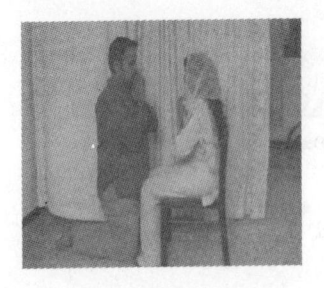

Half rise yourself. Repeat mentally "I thank you for being here. I ask your personality to step aside. I ask your higher self to be in contact with my higher self. Thank you *(here you have to sense the vibrations in your body while watching the 3rd Eye Chakra).*

Pick up the cymbals lying on the mat on your right hand side next to the chair, with your thumb and index finger.

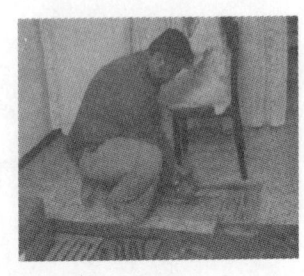

i. Stretch your hands. Place cymbals near to the 3rd Eye Chakra of the student.
ii. Strike cymbals thrice waiting each time for the vibrations to finish.
(Note : When you strike the cymbals on the 3rd Eye Chakra you have to put the cymbals nearer to both the ears till vibrations end).

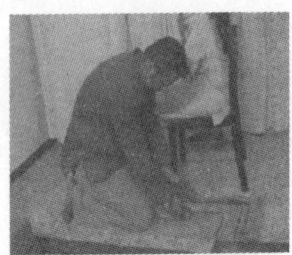

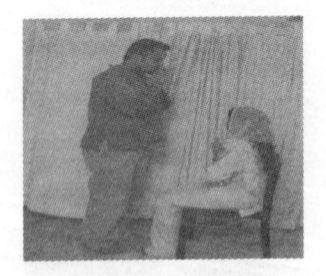

Place cymbals on the mat as before.

Stand up in front of the student.

Take a step to the Right hand side still facing the student and mentally say 'Thank you'

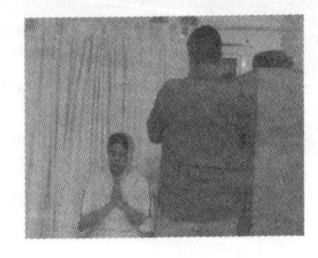

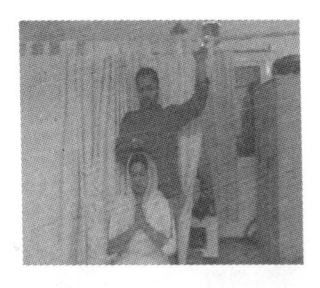

i. Go behind the student.
ii. Place your right hand on the student's head about 2" to 3" away and your left hand high up over your head with palms facing up.
iii. Mentally feel the Reiki energy pass from your left hand to your right hand and on to the Crown Chakra of the student.

i. Point your index and middle finger with the other 3 fingers closed inwards.
ii. Draw "Dai Ku Myo" repeat thrice
iii. Draw "Hon Sha Ze Sho Nain" repeat thrice
iv. Draw "Say Hay Ki" once repeat thrice.

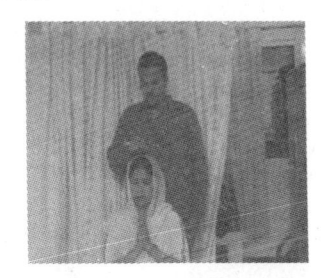

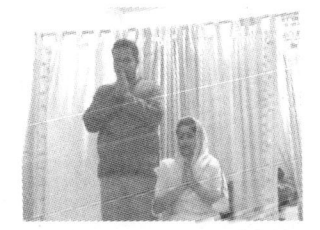

Step on the Right hand side and mentally say "Thank you"

i. Come in front of the student.
ii. Place your Right foot in between the student's feet.

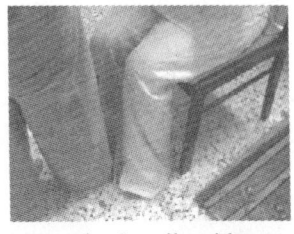

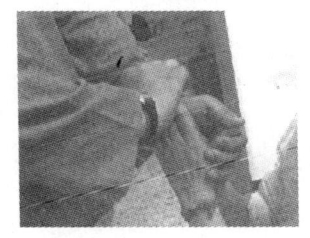

i. Slightly bend and cover student's nails with your right hand.
Note: Your left hand thumb covers both the thumbs of the student.
ii. Put pressure on the nails covered, whilst drawing 'Dai Ku Myo', 'Hon Sha Ze Sho Nain', 'Say Hay Ki' & 'Cho Ku Ray' (on the 3rd Eye)

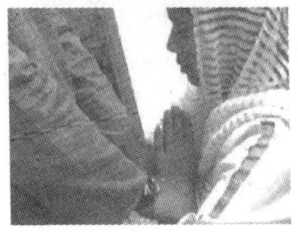

Release hands and catch Wrists. (The small cup technique is completed.

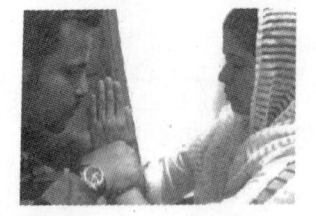

Raise student's hands and blow "Cho" on the Heart Chakra.

Raise student's hands still higher and blow "Ku" on the Throat Chakra

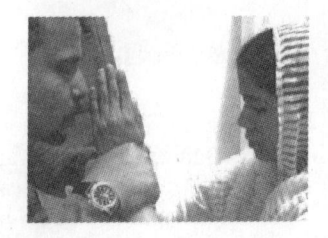

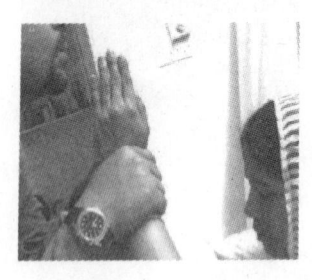

Raise student's hands all the way up and blow "Ray" on the 3rd Eye, whilst bringing students hands on his Crown Chakra. (The breath of Ray should pass between the palms of the student's hands.

Place hands back on chest

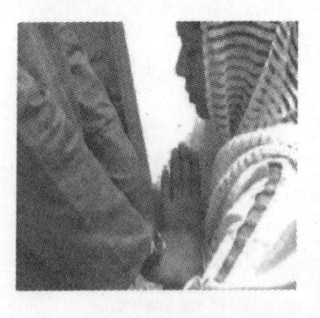

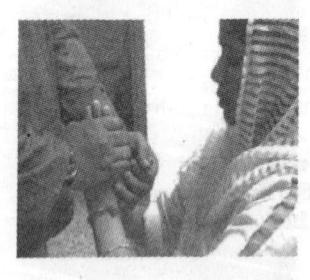

i. Cover both hands of student with your right hand.
ii. Your left thumb covers both the thumbs of the student.
iii. While pressing all the above draw "Dai Ku Myo", "Hon Sha Ze Sho Nain", "Say Hay Ki", "Cho Ku Ray"

i. Release hands and catch wrists.

This completes the Big Cup technique.

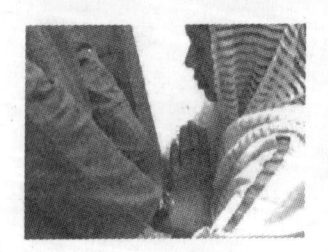

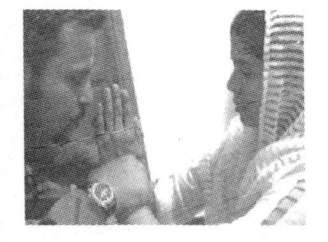

Raise student's hands and blow "Cho" on the Heart Chakra.

Raise student's hands still higher and blow "Ku" on the Throat Chakra

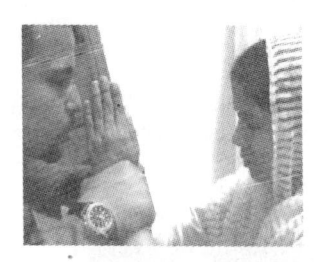

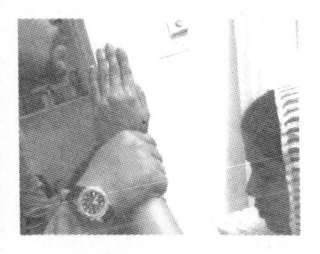

Raise student's hands all the way up and blow "Ray" on the 3rd Eye, whilst bringing students hands on his Crown Chakra. (The breath of Ray should pass between the palms of the student's hands.

Place hands on the chest.

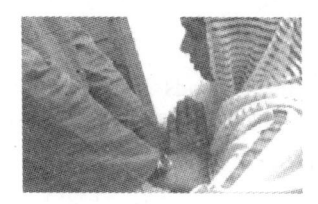

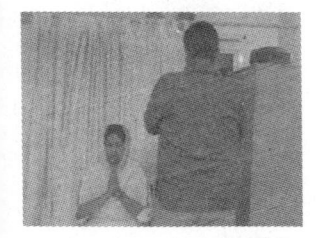

Step on the right hand side and mentally say 'Thank you'

a. Point your index and middle finger with the other 3 fingers closed inwards.
b. Draw "Say Hay Ki" once repeat thrice.

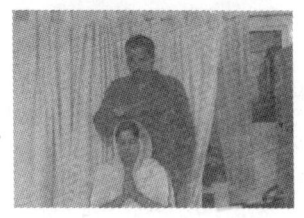

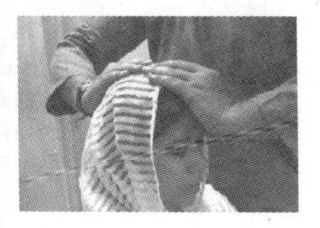

THIS IS AN ATTUNEMENT
1. Look at the picture carefully and take care to press the forehead and back head slightly whilst drawing "Dai Ku Myo", "Hon Sha Ze Sho Nain", "Say Hay Ki", "Cho Ku Ray" once and repeating thrice.

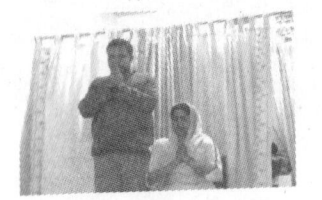

Step on your Right hand side and mentally say "Thank you"

Come in front of the student and place your right foot in between the student's feet.

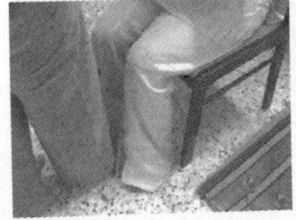

i. Slightly bend and cover student's nails with your right hand.
Note: Your left hand thumb covers both the thumbs of the student.
ii. Put pressure on the nails covered, whilst drawing 'Dai Ku Myo', 'Hon Sha Ze Sho Nain', 'Say Hay Ki' & 'Cho Ku Ray' (on the 3rd Eye)

Place hands back on the chest and catch the student's wrists as shown in the picture.

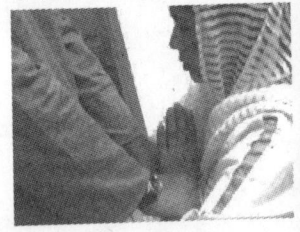

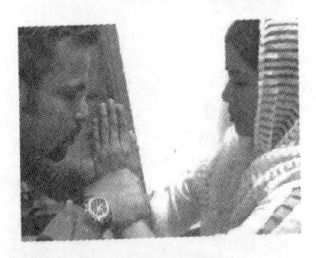

Raise student's hands and blow "Cho" on the Heart Chakra.

Raise student's hands a little higher and blow "Ku" on the Throat Chakra.

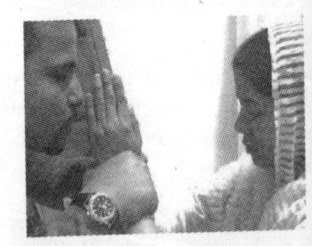

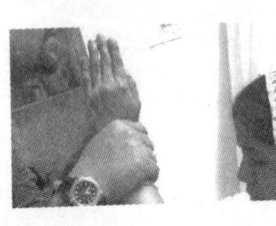

Raise student's hands all the way up and blow "Ray" on the 3rd Eye, whilst bringing students hands on his Crown Chakra. (The breath of Ray should pass between the palms of the student's hands.

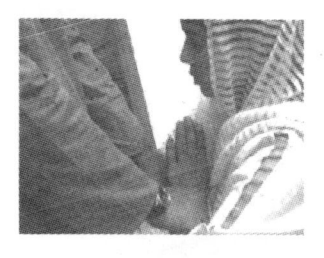

Place student's hands back on the chest.

1. Cover both hands of student with your right hand.
2. Your left thumb covers both the thumbs of the student.
3. While pressing all the above draw "Dai Ku Myo", "Hon Sha Ze Sho Nain", "Say Hay Ki", "Cho Ku Ray"

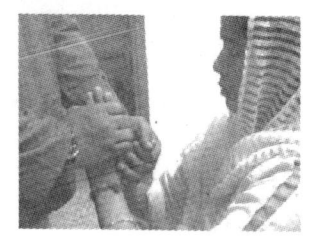

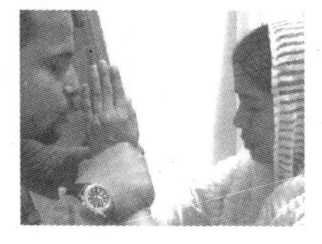

Raise student's hands and blow "Cho" on the Heart Chakra.

Raise student's hands a little higher and blow "Ku" on the Throat Chakra.

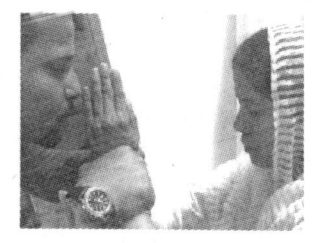

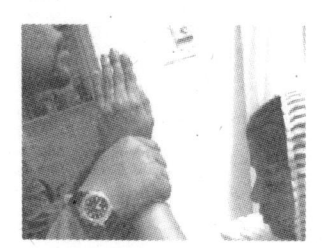

Raise student's hands all the way up and blow "Ray" on the 3rd Eye, whilst bringing students hands on his Crown Chakra. (The breath of Ray should pass between the palms of the student's hands.

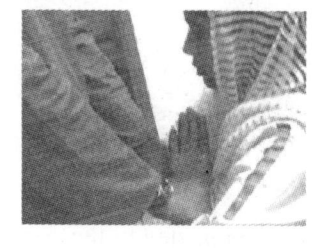

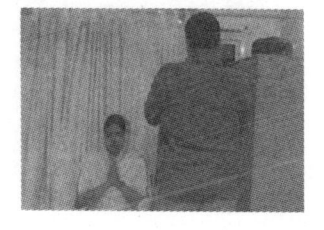

Place hands back on the chest.

Take a step to the right hand side and mentally say "Thank you"

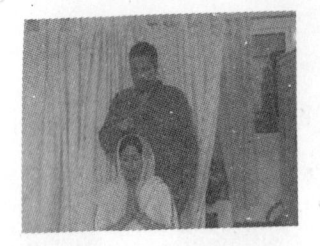

a. Point your index and middle finger with the other 3 fingers closed inwards. Draw "Say Hay Ki" once repeat thrice.

This is an Attunement

1. Both hands cover face, whilst both your thumbs rest on the backside of the skull, behind the ear).
2. Slightly raise the hands upwards drawing all 4 symbols once and repeating thrice.

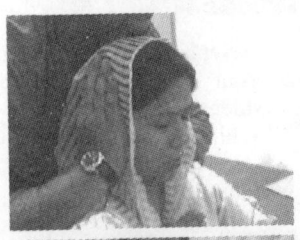

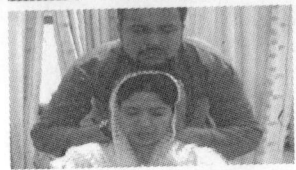

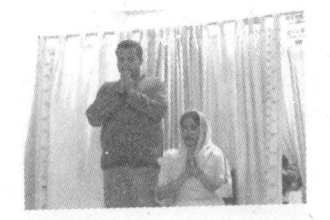

Step on the Right Hand Side and mentally say "Thank you"

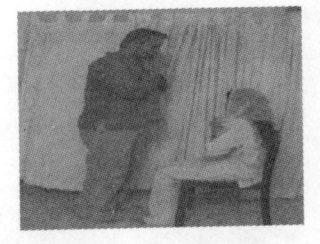

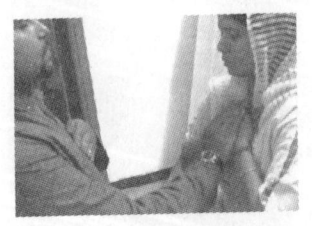

Come and stand in front of the student.

Go on your haunches:
1. Place students hands flat on chest, palms inwards.
2. Place your Right Hand on student's hands
3. Place your Left Hand on your Heart Chakra
4. Draw "Cho Ku Ray" once repeating thrice.

Stand up, step to the right. Join your hands and audibly say "Come back to the room. Now you can open your eyes. Thank you."

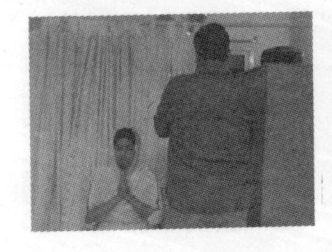

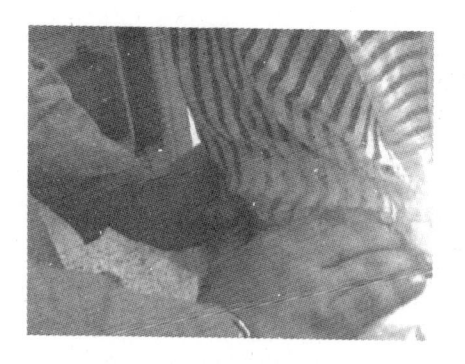

This is an Attunement

NOTE: This is the 2nd Day attunement which is same as Day-1 attunement. All figures from 1 to 46 are to be done but Fig. 47a & 47b are to be replaced by Fig. 52 above.

Description:

(i) Your palms lie on the backside of the student's shoulders.
(ii) Your Right Hand thumb covers the Left Hand thumb (covers the 7th vertebra). Pressurize slightly drawing "Dai Ku Myo", "Hon Sha Ze Sho Nain", "Say Hay Ki", "Cho Ku Ray".

REIKI

3B - THE MASTER / TEACHER
CHAPTER 3

MEDITATION 20 MINUTES

This is what we do. We say, we do not want this, and, do a hundred things to avoid not wanting that. But, if we turn our thinking and attitude and say "I want this" and create a desire to get that, and, do a hundred things to get that, we WILL GET WHAT WE WANT.

Because, out attention is not divided. From negative thoughts we are turning our energy to positive thoughts.

When people visit me, they claim they have diseases, which cannot be healed by the doctors. I tell them with Confidence "You will be cured, I promise you" Then, I immediately encircle them n white light and float them into the air.

Be it high or low blood pressure. Be it Diabetes, Asthma, Arthritis, Rheumatism or any disease, which may take months/years to cure. If you do the healing with compassion, love, patience and honesty - the results will follow quickly.

I repeat again what I have repeated before and will repeat again, "Do lots and lots of visualisation exercises, the clearer the picture, the faster the healing will be"

Now, let's do a 20 minutes meditation.

This will be a simple meditation with the following steps:

1. Sit in your favorite comfortable position or lie down comfortably.
2. Close your eyes.
3. Follow your breath going in and coming out.
4. Follow your breath and listen to the breathing sound.
5. Continue doing the same.
6. While following your breath, listen to your heart beats.

7. Continue doing for the rest of the time.

Open your eyes slowly.

Do these types of exercises 2 to 3 times a day.

REIKI

3B - THE MASTER / TEACHER
CHAPTER 4

WHAT WE HAVE LEARNT SO FAR

I know this in midst of the lesson that I have stopped. But, remember, this is Master's degree. We have to go very slow - Yes, at a snail's pace. The walk of the Tortoise. Safe & sure.

Before we proceed further, we have to ensure that:

1. We have mastered all the Reiki positions.
2. The attunement techniques for Reiki 1.x 2 days, Reiki 2 & Reiki 3A are learnt by heart. We have the mat & the cymbals ready in the attunement room, placed on the Right Hand Side of the chair/wooden stool. The room has been cleansed of negativity for at least 3 days prior to the attunement. We have observed the attunement preparation ourselves.
3. We have meditated and kept a fast as part of preparations.
4. We have to ask ourselves, now that we are Reiki Masters, are we living by the 5 principles of Reiki.
5. What about regression? This is a separate topic by itself. As a Reiki Teacher does not teach regression you have to get acquainted with this technique by taking Hypnotic Therapy classes and ensure that this will include the regression technique.
6. In later chapters in this book we shall discuss some of the problems faced by a Reiki Teacher, which please read and understand carefully.

Shall we continue??

REIKI

3B - THE MASTER / TEACHER
CHAPTER 5

PROBLEMS & PROBLEMS

During the courses held by me, most of the time students revert to me with questions, I have been jotting down their questions and the answers given. I sincerely hope, these will help you to clear May of your doubts.

The first problem faced by me during the attunements was with one of my students by the name of Mr. Pradeep Naik. During the first day of attunements all the 12 students were asked of the experiences in the Attunement room. Whilst 11 of them talked about their experiences excitedly, only one student was quiet, and he said that there were no experiences.

The problem started on the 2nd day, I took Pradeep in the attunement room and whilst giving him the attunement, he felt dizzy. After the attunements were over, he would not get up. Pradeep has a big built; somehow I picked him up and put him on the bed. I tried to revive him and bring him back to consciousness, but he would not come out of it.

I was scared. What to do? What if he dies? All questions come floating to me. What would you do? Call the doctor? Anyway, I sat in a Meditation pose, called on the help of the spiritual guides - Dr. Mikao Usui, Dr. Hayashi, Mrs. Takata & Dr. Pradeep Diwan my Guru, My Teacher. I invoked their help. After about a few minutes pictures started floating up on my mental screen and I was pleased.

After coming back to my conscious level, I got up and kept my Right hand on Pradeep's Crown Chakra, visualized a golden light floating from my Crown Chakra to my Right Hand and whispered softly, "you are coming back in to your body, slowly, visualize I am bringing you back into your body - slow…ly, you are coming back in to you body" and I could see Pradeep's eyes started to flicker, I continued with my whispering that he was coming back to his body, and, after a few minutes his eyes were completely opened and he smiled.

While asking for experiences, Pradeep stated when the last attunement was given to him, he felt something come out of his body and his physical self was just left behind.

Pradeep could see himself and me on the bed from the ceiling in the room. He was floating on the ceiling, Pradeep could also hear me very clearly, but, did not want to return back to the room as he was so happy with this feeling of lightness, this illumination.

The second experiences was with Mr. Rasik Thakker who just leapt out of his body, and, landed up on the ceiling - floating and seeing himself lying down on the ground. When asked how he felt, he said, "I did not want to come back, it's amazing, unbelievable" this has happened when we did the Mind Control Exercise of "Activating your Astral Body"

Similar experience occurred on "Activating your Astral Body" with Dr. Reshma Gurnani, who sat up, but, would not respond to anything being said or instructed to her.

After doing the exercise with her again - special instruction was given "Now you will return to your body fully, your feet, your calves & your thighs have returned and you feel sensations in these areas. You now feel sensations in your hips, Root Chakra, Sexual Chakra, Hara & Solar Plexus. (after a gap) Now, you feel sensations in your chest areas, stomach, shoulders, hands, move your fingers, all the sensations are being return one by one. Your chin, your facial muscles, your forehand all are being activated. You sensations are now fully returned back to you. Your 5 senses are working in their perfect condition. Slow...ly open your eyes"

When Dr. Gurnani opened her eyes, we asked her what had happened, and, she said that though she could hear everything, she could not open her eyes, as they were left out.

There are cases and cases in visual meditation and Reiki, which can never end. But, as I caution you of one thing - NEVER PANIC!! In any situation be calm, if anything goes wrong, please call in your spiritual guides as taught to you in the attunement techniques and request them to help you. Once the Spiritual Guides come to you they will always help you in every phase of your life.

In Visual Exercises, though the ethereal body may leave, this has to return to the physical body - it is only a matter of time, just assume that the person has dozed off to sleep. When the person wakes up, he/she will be in excellent/perfect condition.

Even so for Reiki attunement, most of the experiences the students get are seeing of shadows, colors, out of body experiences, geometrical shapes etc. etc.

Remember, during one of the attunements we are opening up the 3rd Eye Chakra, so these experiences will occur. NOTHING TO WORRY ABOUT OR BE SCARED.

REIKI

3B - THE MASTER / TEACHER
CHAPTER 6

WHAT TO DO AND WHAT NOT TO DO

Questions, Questions & Questions.

≅ **How do we know what is wrong with a person?**

Answer : On placement of hands over the 26 positions of the body, 3 minutes per position, if you concentrate, you will find come across
1. Cold Areas - where you have to do the scooping of bad energy and throw it away in Salt Water
2. Areas where too much energy is being absorbed in to the patients
3. Areas where you feel a slight pain in your hands. These areas are the Problematic areas.

≅ **What to do when I feel & know about the problematic areas?**

The first thing is - you never put this to the patient in a blatant way. You can suggest that while giving Reiki you felt some sort of sensations, which indicate that there is pain in that area/s. Do you have any problems with that area? Ask innocently. If the patient's answer is negative, suggest that he goes to the doctor and gets a medical check up done.

Remember one thing, Reiki is holistic. We are treating the patient on a Mental, Physical & Spiritual level. The problem may still be prevalent on the auric level and the medical science may not be able to prove what we have proved. The pain may attack the physical body from anytime between the days of your giving Reiki up to 6 months period.

REIKI

3B - THE MASTER / TEACHER
CHAPTER 7

VISUAL MEDITATION EXERCISE - THE BALOON & THE STONES

- Seat yourself comfortable on a chair with both your feet touching the ground.
- Do the breathing exercise till you feel you have reached the Alpha Level or feel completely relaxed.
- Visualize someone tying small pebbles on your right hand fingers, which are quite heavy.
- Visualize someone tying balloons on your left hand.
- Keep on doing so till your feel heavy on the right hand and light on the left hand.
- Open your eyes.

RESULTS:

If you see your right hand is lower than your left hand or your left hand is much higher than your right hand - you can classify that your visualization is proper.

Continuous practice of this exercise will help you to succeed with tailor made exercises.

REIKI

3B - THE MASTER / TEACHER
CHAPTER 8

MEDITATION - 20 MINUTES

- Sit in any comfortable position you wish to
- Listen to the sounds around you, the rotating fan, the A/C, birds chirping, people conversing
- Now, listen to your breathing, in-out, in-out, in-out
- Next list to your heart beats
- Mentally try and count the number of different sounds you can hear

Next time you sit for this particular Meditation Exercise try to increase the number of sounds.

REIKI

3B - THE MASTER / TEACHER
CHAPTER 9

WHAT IF NO RESULTS FOLLOW?

Once a student asked me,

"Mr. Mohan what if we complete the course with you, and no results follow?"

This was my reply to the students:

"My class has a maximum of 20 students. If the result is 90%, I consider myself as a failure. During each of my class held over a period of 2 days or approximately 20 hours, special care is taken to follow each student individually, so that no student is left behind. The result is on the second day, at the end of the course, we have a question & answer period, during which an assessment is done on all the students and weak students are pinpointed. These students are requested to come for a refresher course, which is free of charge. Mostly, students do not require coming for more than one refresher course. This ensures that the result if always 100%.

Hence, if the results achieved are always 100% during every training session, the question of "What if NO results follow" does not arise.

During the class session, I never tell the student "We will discuss this later" as it is a known fact that if any question is avoided, there is a chance that the interest of the student may fizzle out. While conversing with any student, eye contact is always maintained. It is a must. That is confidence!

All questions are answered honestly. If the answer is not known, the students are asked to answer that question, if they know the answer.

Students are thus always pleased at the openness and frankness. They know that come whatever may, no wrong teaching will be imparted to them.

Their minds settle down and they feel at ease with themselves and the friendly atmosphere, knowing that whatever they are being taught the teacher knows the subject thoroughly.

REIKI

3B - THE MASTER / TEACHER
CHAPTER 10

THE POSITIVE & THE NEGATIVE MIND

There is a very famous saying

"Ist the Glass half full or half empty"?

The Negative mind will reply - "Half Empty"

whilst the Positive Mind will reply "Half Full"

The first negative taught which rises in your mind is known as an 'elemental'. This taught is smaller that an atom. The main food for this 'elemental' is your negativity. It feeds on your fears - on your doubts - on your anger - on your failures - on all your minus points.

Then the more you dwell on these - the more larger it becomes - the more larger it gets - the more difficult it is for you to crush this taught.

Then - ALL OF A SUDDEN - 'BANGGGG' This same elemental crushes you, sending your head spinning around. Taking you from the heights of success to the bottom rungs of failure.

Whose fault it is anyway "MINE" I would say.
YES - it is you fault if you fail.
YES - it is your fault if you are unsuccessful.
YES - it is your fault if you cannot stand up and say "I am a failure"

Accept things as they are, not as you want them to be. Fight with all the positivity you have in yourself. Tailor make visual exercises to change the taught in your mind from the darkness's of failure and doom to the realms of Light & success. Keep on repeating to yourself the most successful phrase every invented "DAY BY DAY IN EVERY WAY I AM GETTING BETTER AND BETTER AND BETTER"

See the improvement in yourself. While looking into the mirror each morning do not frown but smile and wish yourself "A very happy GOOD MORNING"

See yourself flying through the day successfully. Be a Positive person - be SUCCESSFUL.

REIKI

3B - THE MASTER / TEACHER
CHAPTER 11

WHY IS A CERTIFICATE NECESSARY?

That's simple.

How can you differentiate between a fake teacher and a genuine teacher?

The colorization of each certificate given is separate.

The Reiki 1 Certificate is Blue in Color
The Reiki 2 Certificate is Green in Color
The Reiki 3A & 3B Certificates are Red in Color with a golden label on the Left Hand Side.

No doubt these can be forged. But, ask your sub-conscious mind - have I tried hard to get this Certificate? What's the difference between the Genuine Teacher and the Fake Teacher.

Well, the Fake Teacher can always live in fear of being caught. But, the Genuine Teacher is never frightened. A Genuine Teacher is at peace within himself, which over the years reflects in his face, which glows with happiness.

The Genuine Teacher looks at the Certificate with Pride and a sense of Achievement whilst the Fake Teacher looks at the Certificate with shame, knowing deep within himself that he is a cheat.

BE PROUD OF YOURSELF - WORK HARD AT WHAT YOU WANT TO ACHIEVE AND FEEL THE DIFFERENCE.

REIKI

3B - THE MASTER / TEACHER
CHAPTER 12

LET'S SUM UP

Once more. We sum up.

We have learnt how to handle the problems. Are you more confident about yourself? No?! Read the Chapter 8 of Book 3B again, you are protected by the spiritual guides. Nothing ever will go again, this is the only assurance I can give you.

What goes up comes down. Any student of yours having an O.B.E. (Out of body experience) will have to return to the body, in a matter of time.

Remember also that attunements are given once in a lifetime. Never repeat the attunements again.

Students coming to you fresh will get the attunements from you, whilst students coming to you who have done Reiki from another Teacher, will not be given attunements for that particular level. So, it is not necessary to charge fees from that student for it will be a Refresher course for this student.

If you even have a problem you can write to me on any of the address given above - (e-mail, hot-mail, postal or can also call me on the phone)

I wish you all the best and pray that you be a success at whatever you do that is positive and clean.

REIKI

3B - THE MASTER / TEACHER
CHAPTER 13

THE PRESENTATION OF THE CERTIFICATES

THE JAPANESE TRADITION

After each course in Reiki is over, the teacher and the students stand in a circle and chant "OM" three times.

After which the teacher calls the name of each student individually. The student comes and stands in front of the teacher.

The teacher bows down from the waist and the student repeats the gesture. The Certificate is then presented to the student and they again bow from waist downwards.

This is a usual procedure while presenting the certificate.

REIKI

3B - THE MASTER / TEACHER
CHAPTER 14

HOW TO CLOSE EACH DAY

THE BEAR HUG

During the end of each session (every day) the Reiki Teacher and the students stand in a round circle, entwine their hands and chant "OM" three times.

After the chanting of the "OM" the Reiki Teacher hugs each student individually, whilst all the students hug each other also.

This brings to end the current day's session.

Only to meet another day.

REIKI

3B - THE MASTER / TEACHER
CHAPTER 15

QUESTIONS

The most proper questions to be asked will be on the following lines :

1. Now that I have completed the full book - can I declare myself as a REIKI MASTER?

Answer : Yes, by completing this courser, you are not only a Reiki Master, but also, you are in a level above the Reiki Masters - YOU ARE A REIKI TEACHER - AN INDEPENDENT TEACHER OF REIKI. CONGRATULATIONS.

2. Can I start my own classes?

Answer : Yes, provided you feel confident yourself. Ask your sub conscious mind "Have I done justice to this course? Have I practiced the norms in the book? Do I live with the attitude of Gratitude? Have I mastered the Symbols? Have I mastered the art of giving Attunements? If your answer to each of the above is "YES" Well, go ahead and start your own classes.

3. I have received the Certificates for Rciki I, Reiki 2 & Reiki 3A which proves that I have done the course sincerely, but, what about the Teacher's Certificate?

Answer : Sorry, till you do not come in my presence and I do not see you give attunements without referring to the book, I cannot present this Certificate to you. If you can enroll for a Certificate with me on the internet - on my travels I can call you to visit me - where a test will be given - if you succeed a Certificate will be issued immediately on payment of US$150/-. (My Internet address is mentioned in the book)

4. When can you visit us?

Answer : It depends on my itinerary. You will be given ample notice to be free during that time. The date/time will be advised to you on your e-mail or by fax. If you delay or are late due to what so ever the reasons - the appointment will be canceled.

5. Will you be giving us attunements for all the 3 levels during you visit?

Answer : No, the Certificates issued to you were assessed on your experiences while you received the attunements from your partner. If they were fictitious, it is your doing. But, if they were genuine, you do not need another attunement. These are only given once in a life span.

6. What if we want only the attunements?

Answer : Sorry, this cannot be done. You have to attend a proper course, which is conducted on regular basis.

7. What if we want to attend your course?

Answer : Please write to me on my e-mail or hotmail address and we shall revert. My regular class fees are :

Reiki Course 1 - US$25/- - 2 days course from 9.00 am to 5.00 p.m. each day
Reiki Course 2 - US$50/- 2.1/2 days course
Reiki Masters 3A - US$100/- 5 hours course. It is must for students to attend and practice Reiki 1 & 2 courses on repeated regular course to get a hang of the full course and Reiki positions plus should be in a position to answer questions posited by the students.

8. What is your itinerary?

Answer : Depends on response of each territory.

9. Now that I have purchased this book, what should I do?
Answer : This book is unique. Every book in the market has a serial No. Here is what you do.

a. Tear off the perforated first page - fill it up and post is to us. Ensure all sections are completely filled.

b. After each Reiki Degree is complete, we can provide you with a Reiki Certificate subject to your answers being satisfactory. Else, we give you 2 additional chances. After which your fee will be refunded minus US$5/- which should be postage charges.

c. If all the answers are right, the Certificate will be posted to you within 21 days.

d. You will automatically be advised of my visit to your territory. If you wish to have the Master/Teachers Certificate please let us know in advance.

REIKI

3B - THE MASTER / TEACHER
CHAPTER 16

JUST TO SAY GOOD-BYE:

Dear Reader,

Hope you have enjoyed this book. The purpose is living with the family and living with spiritualism, gathering least of Karmas to get Nirvana.

Let's do one exercise.

- DO A GOOD DEED TO AN UNKNOWN PERSON.

- DO NOT ASK BACK FOR A FAVOUR OR A THANK YOU.

- REQUEST THE PERSONE TO PASS ON THIS GOOD DEED TO ANOTHER NEEDY PERSON.

- THIS PERSON PASSES THE GOOD DEED TO SOMEONE ELSE.

- AND SO ON.

- LET'S FORM A CHAIN   WHAT YOU GIVE ALWAYS RETURNS.

- MAY BE JUST MAY BE WE WILL GET BACK WHAT WE HAVE GIVEN WHEN WE NEED IT MOST?

REIKI

3B - THE MASTER / TEACHER
CHAPTER 17

THE HUMAN ANATOMY

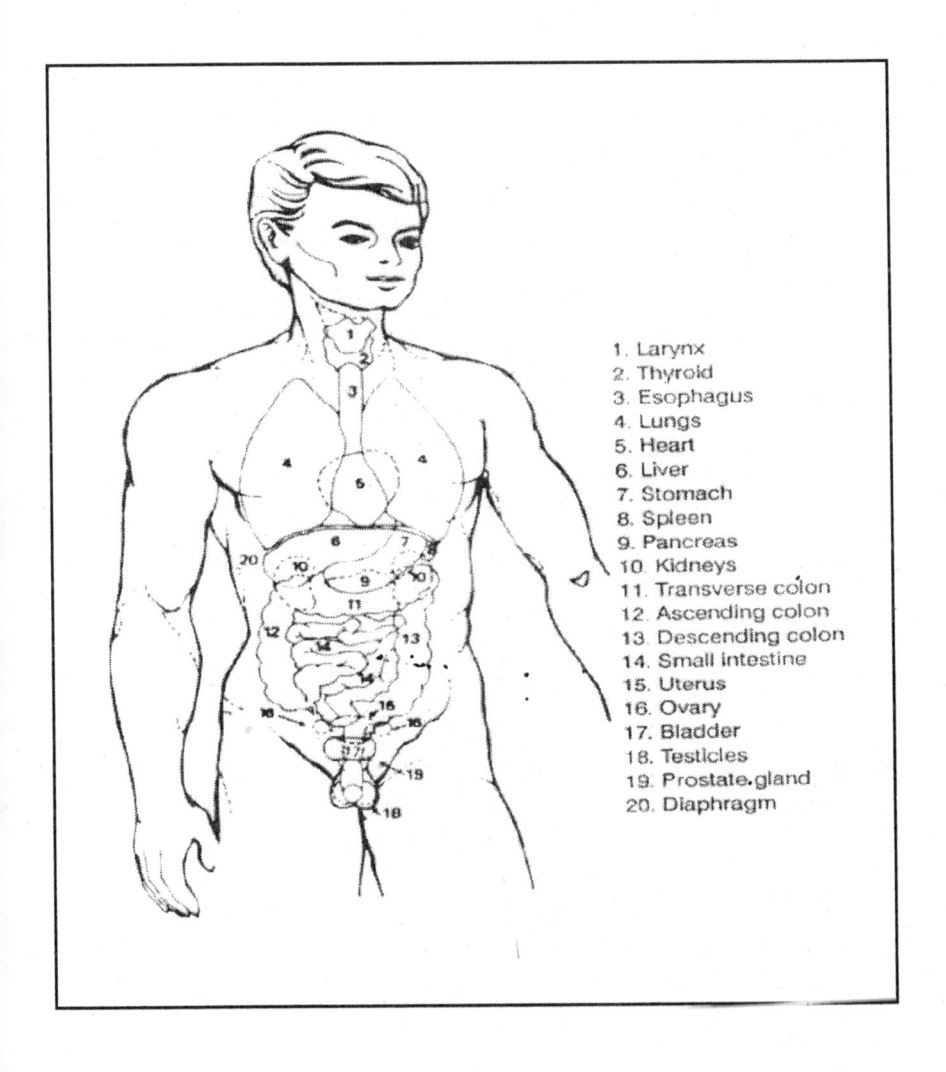

1. Larynx
2. Thyroid
3. Esophagus
4. Lungs
5. Heart
6. Liver
7. Stomach
8. Spleen
9. Pancreas
10. Kidneys
11. Transverse colon
12. Ascending colon
13. Descending colon
14. Small intestine
15. Uterus
16. Ovary
17. Bladder
18. Testicles
19. Prostate gland
20. Diaphragm

REIKI

3B - THE MASTER / TEACHER
CHAPTER 18

DISEASES & HAND POSITIONS FOR TREATMENTS

1. Anemia — Sweeping, Full Body Reiki front & Back
2. Anxiety — Sweeping, Full Body Reiki Once a day
3. Appendicitis — Sweeping Heart, Solar Plexus, Hara, Liver Front & Heart, Solar Plexus, Hara, Kidneys, Root on the back. + giving Reiki on the same positions Front & Back.
4. Arthritis — Full body sweeping, group healing of full body, about 4 to 6 months minimum.
5. Asthma on — Sweeping Head to Hara. Front Side Reiki Eyes, Temples, Ears, Front & Back of Head, Back of Head, Front & Back of Neck, Thymus/Thyroid, Heart, Solar Plexus. Back Side Reiki on Thymus/Thyroid, Heart, Solar Plexus & Root.
6. Autism — Sweeping, Full body Reiki twice a day, probably Marathon or Group Healing. Only 30 to 40% improvement can be found in such cases.
7. Bed Wetting — Full body.
8. Bladder Stones — Sweeping Heart, Solar Plexus, Hara, Liver Front & Heart, Solar Plexus, Hara, Kidneys, Root on the back. + giving Reiki on the same positions Front & Back.
9. Blood Pressure High — Sweeping & Full Body
10. Blood Pressure Low — Sweeping & Full Body
11. Brain Tumor — Group Healing or Marathon Reiki till results follow
12. Bronchitis — Sweeping Head to Hara. Front Side Reiki on Eyes, Temples, Ears, Front & Back of Head, Back of Head, Front & Back of Neck, Thymus/Thyroid, Heart, Solar

	Plexus. Back Side Reiki on Thymus / Thyroid, Heart, Solar Plexus & Root
13. Burns	Excessive sweeping & aura cleaning, Medipic Technique & full Reiki without touching the body
14. Chest Infection	Sweeping Head to Hara. Front Side Reiki on Eyes, Temples, Ears, Front & Back of Head, Back of Head, Front & Back of Neck, Thymus/Thyroid, Heart, Solar Plexus. Back Side Reiki on Thymus/Thyroid, Heart, Solar Plexus & Root.
15. Chicken Pox	Excessive sweeping to stop itching, full Reiki, preferably Group healing twice a day.
16. ChildBirth Complications	Heart, lower positions front & back at least 3 to 4 times a day
17. Cholera	Sweeping of complete body, full Reiki thrice a day.
18. Coma	Sweeping, marathon Reiki at least 8 hours daily.
19. Common Cold	Sweeping Head to Hara. Front Side Reiki on Eyes, Temples, Ears, Front & Back of Head, Back of Head, Front & Back of Neck, Thymus/Thyroid, Heart, Solar Plexus. Back Side Reiki on Thymus/Thyroid, Heart, Solar Plexus & Root.
20. Conjunctivitis	Sweeping on eyes. First 5 positions on the front side, heart front & back, Root front & back.
21. Constipation	Heart, Front & back lower Chakras
22. Convulsions	Excessive sweeping of full body. Head positions minimum 5 minutes each, heart, solar & root front & on the back Heart, Solar & Root.
23. Dandruff	Sweeping of Crown Chakra, Reiki front side on all 5 positions of the head, Heart

24. Deafness	front & back, Solar & Root Sweeping of Crown Chakra, Reiki front side on all 5 positions of the head, Heart front & back, Solar & Root
25. Dehydration	Sweeping, Heart & Lower Chakras front & back.
26. Depression	Look out for energy leak, stick from sexual chakra to feet, to armpits to hands to shoulders and crown, come back to the other side of the body, finishing at the starting point. Then full body Reiki. Within 21 days depression should vanish.
27. Diabetes	Excessive sweeping on the lower chakras front & back. Minimum 10 minutes on Solar Plexus, Hara, Liver/Pancreas for front side of the body and on the back side Solar Plexus, Hara, Kidneys & Root 10 minutes each. Preferable group healing.
28. Diarrhea	Excessive sweeping on the lower chakras front & back. Minimum 10 minutes on Heart, Solar Plexus, Hara, Liver/Pancreas for front side of the body and on the back side Heart, Solar Plexus, Hara, Kidneys & Root 10 minutes each. Preferable group healing.
29. Dysentary	Sweeping of the lower Chakras. Front Reiki on Solar Plexus, Hara, Liver, Spleen/Pancreas, Spermitical Cords, Back Reiki on Solar Plexus, Hara, Root, Kidneys
30. Epilepsy	Excessive sweeping of the full body, Marathon Group healing minimum 8 hours daily for over 3 months can improve condition of the patient tremendously.
31. Flat Foot	Reiki on only Chakras & feet front & back
32. Flu	Sweeping Head to Hara. Front Side Reiki on Eyes, Temples, Ears, Front & Back of Head, Back of Head, Front & Back of

	Neck, Thymus/Thyroid, Heart, Solar Plexus. Back Side Reiki on Thymus/Thyroid, Heart, Solar Plexus & Root.
33. Frozen Shoulder	Sweeping on painful areas, Reiki on full head positions, front & back of the neck, thymus thyroid, shoulder joints, heart for front side of the body. For back side, shoulders, thymus thyroid, heart, solar plexus & root 3 minutes per position minimum 3 months.
34. Gastritis	Sweeping Head to Hara. Front Side Reiki on Eyes, Temples, Ears, Front & Back of Head, Back of Head, Front & Back of Neck, Thymus/Thyroid, Heart, Solar Plexus. Back Side Reiki on Thymus/Thyroid, Heart, Solar Plexus & Root.
35. Growing Pains	Full body Reiki.
36. Headaches	Depends of what type. Cover affected areas.
37. Heart Burn	Sweeping Head to Hara. Front Side Reiki on Eyes, Temples, Ears, Front & Back of Head, Back of Head, Front & Back of Neck, Thymus/Thyroid, Heart, Solar Plexus. Back Side Reiki on Thymus/Thyroid, Heart, Solar Plexus & Root.
38. Heart Diseases	Same as '37'.
39. Hiccups	Sweeping of Front & Back of Neck Chakra. Reiki on Thymus/ Thyroid,
40. HIV Infection	Excessive sweeping, burning of auras, creating new auras, chakra balancing & then Marathon Reiki.
41. Hypertension	Full Body Reiki.
42. Hysteria	Group Healing
43. Impotence	Sweeping of the lower Chakras. Front Reiki on Solar Plexus, Hara, Liver, Spleen/Pancreas, Spermitical Cords, Back Reiki on Solar Plexus, Hara, Root,

	Kidneys
44. Indigestion	Full body Reiki
45. Influenza	Sweeping Head to Hara. Front Side Reiki on Eyes, Temples, Ears, Front & Back of Head, Back of Head, Front & Back of Neck, Thymus/Thyroid, Heart, Solar Plexus. Back Side Reiki on Thymus/Thyroid, Heart, Solar Plexus & Root.
46. Insomnia	The first 5 positions, Heart, Solar Plexus on the front side of the body, and, on the back side. Heart and Solar Plexus.
47. Insanity	Marathon Reiki
48. Irritable Bowel Syndrome	Front side of the body Heart, Liver, Pancreas/Spleen, Solar Plexus, Hara & on the back side, Heart, Solar Plexus and Hara.
49. Jaundice	Marathon group healing.
50. Kidney Stones	Excessive sweeping on the Kidneys and Reiki. 30 minutes on the Kidneys area, plus back Solar Plexus, Hara.
51. Laryngitis	Reiki on 3rd Eye, Throat front & back, Heart, Solar Plexus on the back side Thymus Thyroid.
52. Lungs Collapsed	Full body Reiki Marathon Group.
53. Malaria	Full body Reiki Marathon Group.
54. Measles	Full body Reiki group healing.
55. Menopause	Sweeping of the lower Chakras. Front Reiki on Solar Plexus, Hara, Liver, Spleen/Pancreas, Spermitical Cords, Back Reiki on Solar Plexus, Hara, Root, Kidneys.
56. Mumps	Reiki on 3rd Eye, Throat front & back, Heart, Solar Plexus on the back side Thymus Thyroid.
57. Muscle Contractions	Excessive sweeping of full body, full body Reiki till patient feels relaxed minimum 21 days.
58. Muscle Cramps	Excessive sweeping of full body, full body

	Reiki till patient feels relaxed minimum 21 days.
59. Nausea	Full body Reiki.
60. Nose Bleed	Eyes, 3rd Eye Chakra, back head chakra.
61. Osteoarthritis	Excessive sweeping, Group Healing.
62. Piles	Sweeping of the lower Chakras. Front Reiki on Solar Plexus, Hara, Liver, Spleen/Pancreas, Spermitical Cords, Back Reiki on Solar Plexus, Hara, Root, Kidneys.
63. Pimples	On affected area - Reiki.
64. Pneumonia	Sweeping Head to Hara. Front Side Reiki on Eyes, Temples, Ears, Front & Back of Head, Back of Head, Front & Back of Neck, Thymus/Thyroid, Heart, Solar Plexus. Back Side Reiki on Thymus/Thyroid, Heart, Solar Plexus & Root.
65. Pregnancy	Sweeping of the lower Chakras. Front Reiki on Solar Plexus, Hara, Liver, Spleen/Pancreas, Spermitical Cords, Back Reiki on Solar Plexus, Hara, Root, Kidneys
66. Sciatica	Reiki on Root Chakra with excessive sweeping.
67. Sexual Weakness	Sweeping of the lower Chakras. Front Reiki on Solar Plexus, Hara, Liver, Spleen/Pancreas, Spermitical Cords, Back Reiki on Solar Plexus, Hara, Root, Kidneys.
68. Sinusitis	Sweeping Head to Hara. Front Side Reiki on Eyes, Temples, Ears, Front & Back of Head, Back of Head, Front & Back of Neck, Thymus/Thyroid, Heart, Solar Plexus. Back Side Reiki on Thymus/Thyroid, Heart, Solar Plexus & Root.
69. Sleep Walking	Full body Reiki.
70. Spondylitis	Excessive Sweeping, back side Throat, Thymus/Thyroid, Heart, Solar Plexus,

71. Stomach Disorders	Hara & Root. Sweeping of the lower Chakras. Front Reiki on Solar Plexus, Hara, Liver, Spleen/Pancreas, Spermitical Cords, Back Reiki on Solar Plexus, Hara, Root, Kidneys.
72. Stress	Full body Reiki.
73. Sun Burn	Full body Reiki keep hands about 2" to 3" away from the body.
74. Tinnitus	The first 5 positions of the body - Reiki.
75. Trauma	Group Healing.
76. Tubercullosis	Group Healing - Full body Reiki.
77. Typhoid	Group Healing Full body Reiki.
78. Vertigo	Group Healing Full body Reiki.
79. Vision Blurred	The first 5 positions of the body - Reiki.
80. Vomiting	Excessive sweeping from Crown to Heart & Reiki on the first 5 positions, front & back of the neck, Thymus/Thyroid, Heart.
81. Women's Ailments	Sweeping of the lower Chakras. Front Reiki on Solar Plexus, Hara, Liver, Spleen/Pancreas, Spermitical Cords, Back Reiki on Solar Plexus, Hara, Root, Kidneys.

FORTHCOMING BOOKS in the MAGIC SERIES BY Dr. Mohan Makkar Ph.D. (A.M.):

- **Health Magic** — Ingredients from the kitchen are used to treat dozens of diseases. No ill effects. Easy to follow recipes. Indexed. Ingredients marked in English/Hindi.

- **The Magic Of Archangels** — The bible says that Archangels are given to every human born on earth, they are there to help you. Do you have them? Follow the book and look at the changes in your life.

- **Rudraksh Magic** — Every one wants a Rudraksh. But, how do you know this is a genuine Ruraksh or a fake one? What is the Mantra of each Rudraksh? How does it effect the one wearing it?

- **Breath Magic** — No body learns how to breathe when one is born. Why the illnesses? What are the breathing exercises in Yoga and other institutions. Easy to follow breathing exercises. Do away with the daily morning walk. Feel energetic throughout the day.

- **Acupressure Magic** — Akin to Acupuncture. Learning easy to do exercises just by pressing some points in your body. Feel the difference in your day to day health.

- **Feng Shui Magic** — Feeling out of balance with your life? At home with your spouse, with children. Unwanted arguments, financial difficulties? Did you check your house for the 'Chi' 'Ki' 'Prana' if it is balanced. Does the negative energy have a way to get out? Easy to follow steps to a new magical tomorrow.

- **Chakra Magic** — a study of Chakras in different societies in various countries. Transcedental Meditation, Radhaswami, Zen Buddhism etc. Learn the intricacies of Chakra Magic and studies made by the veterans.

- **Spiritual Story Magic** — Heart touching stories collected from different corners of the globe. A story a day, will make you cry from inside out and teach you a spiritual lesson. Do good to one guy every day, do not expect anything back, but, tell to guy to pass it on. One day, maybe, that good will bounce back to you. Wanna challenge?

- **Symbollogy Magic** — Dozen of symbols to draw on your main door, put as an amulet, draw on the walls of your house to bring good luck, evade of evil, bring peace, prosperity etc.

- **Shirdi Sai Bhajans** — why these difficulties in life? Should I ask the lord to give me what I do not have? But, why, he knows everything. Doubts removed in a melodious way by rendering everything at the feet of His Holiness Sri Satchitanand Sai Baba of Shirdi.

- **Hindi poems** — not in the pure Hindi language as written by the Aacharyas and Hindi Pandits. But, simple Hindi asking for peace and solace to live life as life should be lived.